SMALL WONDER

SMALL WONDER

the story of a child born too soon

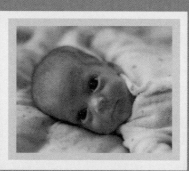

SUSAN LASCALA

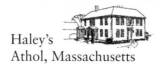

Haley's
Athol, Massachusetts

Haley's
Post Office Box 248
Athol, Massachusetts 01331
haley.antique@verizon.net
1.800.215.8805

Edited by Marcia Gagliardi and Jane P. Gagliardi, M.D.
Copy edited by Mary-Ann DeVita Palmieri with bg Thurston.

Cover design by Abigail Rorer.
Cover photograph by Susan LaScala.

With thanks to Mike Ruocco.

Thanks to Alfred Publishing Company, Van Nuys, California, for permission on pp. 153-154 to use the lyrics to "Love Is a Very Light Thing" from the musical *Fanny*, 1954, with music and lyrics by Harold Rome.

Printed by the Highland Press.

Library of Congress Cataloging-in-Publication Data
LaScala, Susan.
  Small wonder : the story of a child born too soon / Susan LaScala.
    p. cm.
  Includes bibliographical references and index.
  ISBN 978-1-884540-79-0
  1. Blomstedt, Sarah--Health. 2. Premature infants--United States--Biography. 3. Neonatal intensive care. I. Title.
  RJ253.5.B66 2008
  618.92'0110092--dc22
  [B]
                              2007047942

To the babies and those who care for them.

It is a fearsome thing to love what death can touch.
—words from a New England tombstone

CONTENTS

A VERY SPECIAL NEWBORN

a foreword by Barbara Wolk Stechenberg, MD

Twenty-two years ago when Sarah Blomstedt, first called simply Baby LaScala, unexpectedly decided to make her appearance in the world, babies of her size and prematurity faced a grim forty percent survival rate. Those who did survive often experienced long-term problems related to their early births. Even now, with advances made in the care of premature babies, infants the size Sarah was at birth have a mortality rate of twenty percent. They can still have many potential long-term problems.

When Sarah was born, neonatology itself was in its infancy. Many neonatal intensive care units were only ten or so years old. Today, the world of neonatology changes constantly. Pediatric residents, physicians learning to become pediatricians, joke about returning to the NICU after a six-month hiatus and finding that everything has changed. The field evolves that quickly.

Despite new technology with its tubes, special intravenous feeding, and other bells and whistles, there are still many risks faced by premature babies. The most common of these risks is infection. Very small premature infants have under-developed immune systems. Most importantly, they lack the natural barrier of the thicker skin that full-term infants have to help fight off infections. This makes them even more vulnerable to infection from germs that normally just stay on the surface of the skin.

One invasive germ causes yeast infections. When Sarah developed her yeast infection, there were only a few reports from other medical centers about this special problem. To have a yeast infection clog up both kidneys and prevent the normal escape route for urine to rid the body of wastes was (and is) extremely rare. To add irony, her father is a kidney doctor.

All of us—medical personnel and Sarah's family—felt as though we were making it up as we went along as we figured out what to do to encourage Sarah to survive. We were so fortunate to have a team of nurses, doctors, and parents who were willing to try anything for Sarah.

But what about Sarah? It is hard to convey how very special she was. After reading the draft of Susan's book, I was in the NICU seeing another infant and ran into David, Sarah's primary care nurse so many years ago. I had only to mention one word about this book and he immediately remembered Sarah, her family, and her stay in the unit. I asked him how, after taking care of hundreds of premature infants in the intervening twenty years, he could remember her vividly. He shrugged in his humble way—she was different. So feisty! So bursting with life! She had been as cute as the button-like hemangioma on her forehead.

Sarah's dad, Jeff, told me Susan was writing a memoir about Sarah and that he could not read it because he did not want to re-live those excruciating days and nights. I myself remembered being scared to death about Sarah and her chances the whole summer after she was born, and I wondered if I could manage to read the manuscript. I was hesitant when Susan asked me. Furthermore, it is always difficult to see yourself mirrored in other people's eyes. As physicians we are programmed, at least on one level, to present ourselves as confident and poised. Ordinarily, we don't have to read a patient or parent account of how we behaved during a difficult time.

Curiosity eventually got the better of me, however, after Susan gave me her writing. She enticed me with a few chapters, and I knew I had to see the whole thing. With Kleenex box in hand on a private stretch of Cape Cod beach, I read the draft. My older daughter was with me and wondered what I was reading that made tears stream down my face.

"What happened to the baby? Why are you crying?" It was difficult to explain—some were tears of joy for how well Sarah did in the face of such significant problems, but mainly, they were tears of appreciation.

Susan had given me a gift, a rare glimpse into two worlds. One is the world of intensive care nurses. Whether in the neonatal or pediatric ICU, the job they do is incredible. As a physician who is a consultant in both units and may spend a few hours there each day, I certainly have had a healthy respect for their role. Reading this book, however, and seeing the relationship that the nurses built with this family made me understand, even more, how they truly are the primary caregivers. But what affected me most profoundly was the opportunity to see the experience of Sarah's first year through Susan's eyes.

As physicians, we may feel we are empathetic and caring, but we really have no idea the emotional roller coaster many of our parents are riding. Nor can we understand all the pressures that they feel and all the worries they encounter both inside and outside the walls of the hospital.

Susan's story of her daughter Sarah's first challenging year brings us along on the roller coaster. Reminding us again and again of the potentials, mysteries, and strengths of the human body and human spirit, *Small Wonder* is a unique story by an incredible mother about her extraordinary child.

BABY LASCALA

The nurse's aide wheeled me down the corridor. She hadn't said a word when she pulled the wheelchair up to my bedside. Instead, the nurse had done all the talking as she helped me out of bed. "Okay, here we go . . . carefully. Here, let me get the IV. Turn . . . turn . . . there." Gingerly, I let my bottom settle onto the seat of the wheelchair. The nurse organized my IV tubing and pulled in the loose ends of my johnny. She released the hand brake on each wheel, and then there was a moment of silence. What could she say? "Good luck?" or "Have a good visit?" Finally, she went with, "We'll see you in a little while." She placed a light hand on my shoulder, then turned away. The silent aide took it from there.

After a ride down a long hallway, we turned a corner. I saw the sign: Neonatal Intensive Care Unit. The aide punched a button on the wall and double doors opened. She pushed my chair through the doors into an anteroom, past sinks, and then through another door. A woman sitting at the desk looked at me, looked at the aide, looked at me again, and nodded, her eyes and a slight tilt of her chin directing my driver. Rolling between rows of Plexiglas boxes, the wheelchair moved into the room. We continued forward, approaching a place where a crowd of green backs and legs formed a solid wall.

The group huddled around the warmer as if hiding a big secret. Then one face turned to look at me. The young man turned back and spoke to his colleagues. The wall parted and the bodies moved politely— almost apologetically—aside to open a space in front of a waist-high table. I looked up at the people in scrubs, and the faces looked down at me. None of us attempted any amenities. Feeling very small, I placed my hands on the wheels and inched my chair closer. I could not get up out of the wheelchair. The layers of my belly felt as if they were just barely held together by staples I'd heard snapping into my skin the night before, and my freedom was limited by the length of the IV tubing. Unable to stand, I craned my neck to see the surface of the table.

A tiny creature lay on the open warmer. It did not look like a baby, not even like a miniature version of a baby. She was splayed on her back in a position that was totally unnatural for an infant. Newborns usually lie curled up in their cribs, their arms and legs remembering the way they fit in the womb. But this baby's arms stretched flat and straight, and her legs extended and flopped to each side. She lay completely still.

I could not see the baby's face. Bulky white gauze patches covered her eyes to protect them from the bright lights and swallowed her face like a pair of over-sized sunglasses. A white, plastic tube came from her mouth—the endotracheal tube, I knew—and it was attached to the ventilator I could hear breathing in and out, in and out, for her. There was no way to tell what she looked like under the eye patches and the tape that stuck to her cheeks to hold the tube in place—if she had my nose or Jeff's chin. An IV line protruded from her umbilicus, and another came out of a dressing on her arm. The arm was taped to a board to stabilize the IV; the board was just a tongue blade, the wooden stick that the doctor puts on your tongue when he looks down your throat and tells you to say "Ahhhh." All but her head was covered by what looked like the plastic wrap I had in a kitchen drawer. I stared, taking all of it in, but my brain needed a translation of what my eyes were telling me.

A doctor stepped out of the group and introduced himself. He seemed kind and deferential. I asked, "Is that Saran Wrap?" and he responded as if that were an ordinary first question from the mother of a premature baby. Then, in a church-like tone, he gave me my first NICU (short for neonatal intensive care unit) lesson as a parent.

"The baby is wrapped in plastic to minimize fluid loss from her skin," he said, "so she won't become dehydrated. She is in very critical condition as you can see." He took a moment to let that settle. "She is on the warmer because her internal thermostat is still very immature, and it would take too much of her energy to maintain her body temperature in the cool air of the open room." Trying to keep up as he continued the explanations, my thoughts sloshed about.

Restraining themselves from moving for this moment, the strangers in green scrubs hovered around the other side of the table. They were respectfully quiet, like visitors at a wake who avert their eyes when the family members come in to see their loved one.

"She hasn't had much downtime in her first twelve hours," the doctor said. "We connected her to the ventilator for her breathing before she left the delivery room. She's had her blood drawn almost hourly to check her oxygen levels. We had to put IV lines into her arms and umbilical vein to give her fluid and medication."

I moved my eyes back to the warmer. Feeling dazed, I watched a nurse, who could no longer wait to resume her duties, tear another piece of plastic wrap along the serrated metal teeth that lined the box's edge. She placed the box of plastic wrap back on the shelf where it lay in the company of an array of equipment that probably cost as much as a new car, and then she efficiently tucked the second layer of plastic wrap under the baby's neck and around her body as if she were a chicken ready to be put into the fridge.

Turning back to the doctor, I formed the question I hadn't yet asked. "How much does she weigh?"

The doctor said, "Seven hundred nine grams," as if I would understand what that meant. Though I had learned the metric system when I studied pharmacology as a nursing student, 709 grams meant nothing to me when it referred to my baby. I had to ask, "How much is 709 grams?" After a moment of silence, a nurse translated for me: "One pound and nine ounces."

My God, I thought. Is that possible?

I looked at the baby again. I had never seen so small a human, and what I saw in front of me was all foreign and strange. She lay on the heated table under the lights, as if she were an order of fries at McDonald's, was the thought that flitted through my brain. Weird associations jumped out at me, and I felt as if I were on a drug trip, because this little life that lay spread out on the table was so out of my frame of reference that I didn't know how it related to what I had previously known about infants. Nothing about this tiny being resembled the squawking, twenty-four-inch-long boy I had given birth to eighteen months before.

I did not stay in the unit very long. There was nothing for me to do. I knew I couldn't hold the baby and didn't even attempt to touch her. She was covered in plastic, and there was no place to touch. I was an intrusion. She was their baby.

The doctors and nurses were deferential for those first moments. Earlier that day, I'd started grading the hospital staff, and I gave this group an *A* for effort and for giving me a few moments to see my baby. I knew they were trying to keep up with the crisis of the life that lay before them. They acknowledged my right to be there, but they were awkward in my presence. They had work to do.

I took a last look at the tiny being they had labeled "Baby LaScala" on the ID card hanging at the head of the warmer. Then I placed my hands on the wheels and backed the wheelchair away from the table. The nurse's aide took over again. She rolled me along the row of isolettes, through the doors, and out of the unit.

JANUARY 1986

Just twenty-four hours earlier I had been standing in front of
the full-length mirror in my bedroom closet, looking critically at the
pregnant woman who faced me. I hadn't heard my husband walk into the
room, but suddenly his face was above mine in the mirror. He placed his
hands on both sides of my protruding belly and bent to rest his chin on
the top of my head. Our eyes met in the mirror. He grinned.

"You're looking a little frumpy, Dear."

Though Jeff had verbalized my exact thought, I did not smile back at
him. The look that bounced off the mirror and hit him in the face indicated
I did not appreciate the remark, and his grin wilted. He let his hands fall
from my abdomen and slipped out of the room without further comment.

Ten minutes later in my frumpy and rather grumpy state, I moved
around the kitchen and gathered ingredients for breakfast. Sunday
morning pancakes were a family tradition from Jeff's childhood, and I, the
family cook, faithfully carried on the practice. As I measured and mixed
dry ingredients, I reflected on my condition. That morning I'd succumbed
to the requirements of my stretching waistline and climbed into the attic
to retrieve the box of maternity clothes I had worn for the pregnancy with
my son Willie not so long ago. I found no surprises in the box. Pulling
out the tops and pants and the dresses I'd worn to work in the spring
and summer of 1984, I remembered how much fun the maternity outfits
seemed in the early stages of my pregnancy with Willie. The balloon tops
and paneled pants typical of the times represented a new life, a new family,
and I was excited about them. I probably started to wear them even sooner
than I needed to. Now I was dragging the same clothes from the attic for
a surprise pregnancy that came too close to the first, and I was wearing
them two weeks earlier than I had in the first pregnancy because my belly
muscles gave in sooner to the growing baby. Seeing myself in front of the
mirror I thought, well, Susan, you're not exactly glowing.

In spite of how prickly I'd felt in front of the mirror, my dark mood
evaporated in the soothing ordinariness of the Sunday morning routine.
I settled Willie into his high chair and sprinkled a handful of Cheerios on
his tray. Then I collected the rest of the ingredients I needed for pancakes.
After a few minutes of measuring and mixing, I looked down at my waistline
again. Flour dusted the front of the blue and green plaid top I'd chosen
for my first day of maternity wear, and I had to smile at that. I noticed that

my belly kept me farther from the countertop than it had the week before. How far along am I? I calculated as I carried the bowl of batter over to the griddle. About five months and change, I thought. But the dates weren't exactly clear since this pregnancy hadn't exactly been planned.

Taking up a small measuring cup, I scooped batter and poured individual dollops onto the griddle. As they sizzled and then settled into six even rounds, I noticed a feeling below where my waist used to be. I was not uncomfortable—the sensations that traveled across my abdomen were like mild menstrual cramps—but it seemed unusual I would be having them at five months of pregnancy. My due date was April twenty-fourth, and we weren't even halfway through January.

Oh, well, I said to myself for the hundredth time, the second pregnancy is always different from the first. In my work as a nurse practitioner, I said that sentence to patients many times. I believed it when I said it, but I hadn't understood how significant those differences would feel nor how disturbing the changes could be. This pregnancy was definitely a new experience. My thighs had been aching for two weeks. I had been especially uncomfortable the previous day and found myself massaging my upper legs with both hands as I tried to rub out the ache. I felt more tired than I thought I would feel. I recalled that when I was at the same stage of pregnancy with Willie, I was working full-time and feeling terrific. Excited and happy. Energetic, not tired.

I stayed at home with Willie for nine months and then started to work weekends at the UMass Health Center. I wasn't scheduled to work very many hours, and I wasn't worried about working, being pregnant, and taking care of Willie. But in recent days I had found myself feeling a little down, fatigued, uncomfortable in my back and legs more often that not. One day in early January, when the vague symptoms nagged in a low-grade, persistent hum, I phoned my obstetrician's office. The call back came from one of his partners.

"Oh, that sounds pretty normal," he said, dismissing my list of concerns, and I felt silly for calling. I looked at the calendar and thought, I can wait until my routine appointment to talk to my doctor. It's only ten days away.

As I pulled the pancake breakfast together on Sunday, January 12, I was still a few days away from the appointment. The cramps felt wrong. I lifted the edge of a pancake to check the color, then looked over at Willie, who was spreading Cheerios around the tray in front of him. He was exactly eighteen months old that day. Trying to catch the cereal bits before they hit the floor, the dog sat staring at the floor beside him.

"Jeff?" I called out. I wasn't sure where he'd gone after the mirror incident. "The pancakes are ready." Looking sawdusty from whatever project he'd been working on, he walked into the kitchen and kissed me gingerly on the cheek, no doubt concerned about what kind of reception to expect. I smiled, and he looked relieved. He washed his hands, and we sat down at the table together. The rumblings in my abdomen persisted, but they were so mild I wasn't sure they were real, so I didn't say anything about them to Jeff as he poured himself a cup of coffee. We briefly held hands across the table in our rendition of giving thanks, and I smiled at him again as I silently berated myself for having been so humorless in front of the mirror. Then we passed the syrup, picked up knives and forks, and started in on our pancakes.

Our breakfast conversation was mostly nonsensical in that it revolved around Willie, who banged on his tray with a sticky fist and babbled with cheeks full of pancakes. After we finished eating, Jeff took over the kitchen duties, and I walked into the living room to lie down on the carpet. For a few minutes I rested quietly, eyes closed, and soaked up the warm glow emanating from the wood stove. Then I gradually recognized something: there was a rhythm to the cramps. The discomfort started mildly, extended like a belt across my abdomen, then loosened. It happened again. And then again. Out of curiosity I looked at my watch and then closed my eyes. For a few minutes all was quiet, and I allowed my lower back to sink into the floor. The feeling returned. I raised my wrist to eye level and checked the time. I could hear Jeff talking his way through the process of cleaning the syrup off Willie's face before the dog could do the deed. Then I heard the slap of hard shoes on the floor as Willie was set free in the kitchen. In five minutes I felt the tightening again . . . and then five minutes after that.

I opened my eyes and stared upward. We'd been living in the house for a year and a half, and it had problems we were in the process of correcting. One issue was the cathedral ceiling in the living room. It was an imposing barn red. Jeff is the medical director of the local dialysis unit, and in December we had hosted a holiday party for the staff. As we prepared for the party, Jeff said, "Since we are going to change the ceiling to white in January anyway, let's paint something fun on it!"

I was wary. "Like what?" I asked.

"Wait and see," he said.

It was his party, his staff. If he wanted to do something foolish, it was his choice. He went to some trouble to set up scaffolding and painted the words HO! HO! HO! in two-foot-tall white strokes across the red ceiling. A month later, as I lay on the floor staring up at the ceiling, the HO! HO! HO! didn't seem so funny any more.

I was certain this cramping pattern was not normal. The rhythmic cramping and then no cramping was . . . well . . . it was like labor. I lay pressing my back into the floor and thought about it. I was too stunned to move, knowing as soon as I said something to Jeff it would become real. I did not want to break the spell of what had been a nothing-out-of-the-ordinary Sunday morning. Willie played in the kitchen while Jeff ran water in the sink. The dog lay beside me now, chin on paws, and I was about to announce that our quiet life, where ninety minutes earlier the most I had to worry about was how I looked in my maternity clothes, had just gone terribly awry.

SUNDAY'S CHILD IS FULL OF GRACE

White pull-curtains surrounded the hospital bed, but through the mesh at the top I could see a football game. It was playing on every overhead TV in the room. How bizarre, really, on a maternity floor, to have a football game dominating the televisions. I wondered if the game was on for the benefit of the on-call obstetrician or for Jeff and the other fathers-to-be who happened to be stuck in the hospital on a Sunday afternoon. In January of 1986 the New England Patriots had made it to the playoffs, and suddenly everyone was a football fan. At two o'clock in the afternoon we should have been in our living room with Willie sleeping in his crib, Jeff watching the game, and me curled up on the sofa with my feet warming under his thighs. Instead, Jeff whisked Willie across the street to the neighbor's and then drove me to the hospital. A doctor, again not my own but the third partner in the obstetrics practice, worked under a drape that covered the lower half of my body. Feeling fine and even a little silly, I lay on the bed in a time warp. The cramps had been hardly noticeable in the commotion of getting to the hospital. I could hear other activity, seemingly lighthearted and unworried, happening around me and behind the other curtains.

When I heard the obstetrician's muffled words, "The membranes are bulging," I understood I was right to have called him. I had once been on the other end of bulging membranes, and I could imagine what he was seeing. It was in Wenatchee, Washington, in 1982, on a sweltering August evening. I was twenty-six years old and six weeks into my first job as a nurse practitioner. I worked in a community health center serving low-income and migrant farm workers. One Wednesday evening, a name was added to my schedule.

The patient was in the third trimester of her pregnancy with twins. At 6:30 the woman lumbered into the exam room, and I followed with Maria, my exam-room assistant and translator. The patient was Spanish-speaking, and with Maria's help I elicited what history I could. Then, reassuring the woman in English, hoping she might understand my tone if not the words, I helped her into position for the exam. I carefully inserted the warmed metal instrument past her swollen perineum. Looking beyond the moist walls of the woman's vagina, my eyes met something they could not identify at first, something thin, glistening, like a wet, gray balloon. The patient was still more than six weeks from her due date, but when the scene inside the speculum came into focus, I recognized the bulge. It was the membrane that surrounded her babies, pushing out through a soft, ripe cervix that had dilated too early.

Four years later in a hospital in Greenfield, Massachusetts, I lay separated from the rest of the open room by only a thin white curtain, divided from my previous life by bulging membranes. Jeff's attention had been jolted from the football game back to the live action beside him. Though I could hear the crowd roaring behind the doctor's quiet orders and the chatter of the other patients, the sounds of the game no longer mattered. A nurse bustled in and out through the curtains, her cheer suddenly diminished by the turn of events. Then she called an ambulance. For me.

Franklin Medical Center serves the majority of medical needs in our community, but it is a ninety-bed hospital and doesn't have the specialists and equipment needed to care for a woman in preterm labor. I had to be transferred to a larger medical center. While waiting for the ambulance, the doctor asked the nurse to give me an injection of terbutaline, a medication that would stop labor contractions during the forty-five-minute ride to Springfield. The nurse assigned to ride with me in the ambulance said, "You aren't gettin' me in that ambulance till you've had that shot. We don't want to have a baby on Route 91."

A baby? I thought. I just found my maternity clothes this morning. With help from the nurse and the ambulance driver, I moved onto a stretcher. Two EMTs wheeled me down a hall that should have been familiar to me. Willie and I visited Jeff on long workdays when he might not get home before Willie's bedtime. I knew this hallway, but from my horizontal position the hospital seemed foreign. Patients on stretchers see the ceiling, a fact the architects and interior decorators probably don't consider when they choose colors and artwork for the walls. As I thought about that, I began to shiver.

"Ooh, I'm feeling chilled all of a sudden," I said to Jeff through clenched teeth. He walked in long strides next to the stretcher. "It must be the terbutaline." I knew the medication often caused the muscles to tremble.

Jeff hesitated a moment, and then he said, "Uh huh. Probably." But his face said something else, and for the first time since entering the hospital, a place I had allowed myself to imagine would provide a simple resolution of this situation, I saw a waiver in Jeff's bravado.

The ambulance attendants moved my stretcher towards the van at the hospital's emergency-room entrance, and Jeff kissed me a temporary good-bye. Then he stepped back and stood alone, hands in his jacket pockets. He looked a little lost in a place that was usually his domain. He was going home to make arrangements for Willie. Then he would join me at Wesson Women's Hospital.

The ambulance driver and his partner lifted the stretcher up and into the back of the vehicle, a bumpy transfer until the surface under me snapped solidly in place. I felt silly lying down when I was perfectly capable of walking or, at least, of sitting in a wheelchair. The ambulance doors slammed shut, and then there was only the vehicle's movement as it slowly pulled out of the lot. Through the small side window I could see the colors of the ambulance lights bouncing off the cement archway at the ER entrance. Thankfully, the siren remained silent.

The nurse and EMT riding with me knew one another, and they chatted during the speedy ride to Springfield. After a surreal thirty-five minutes, I felt the ambulance slow down. My view was limited, but I thought I recognized the turns as we exited the highway and neared our destination. As the ambulance moved slowly in reverse, the high-pitched beep . . . beep . . . beep told me we had arrived.

The back doors of the ambulance swung open to a zone that, even from my horizontal perspective, looked more like a service entrance than a place for welcoming a new patient. I felt a bit of culture shock. I had left the cheery warmth of our local hospital where everyone knew Jeff as one of their doctors and treated me with special attention as his wife. Less than an hour later, I had landed in the shadow of a large medical center that loomed imperiously over the ambulance and me.

Our arrival time was unfortunate. The change of shift is always a crazy time at a hospital, and I felt the increase in pace as the stretcher bumped and rolled into the old building and a definite lack of warmth from the staff I first encountered. The nurse who had accompanied me in the ambulance patted my shoulder and said, "Good luck, Hon," and the only face I knew disappeared. I lay alone on a stretcher in the dim yellow light of a brown hallway.

My condition didn't seem very urgent any more. I was still shivering under what seemed to be too few blankets, but the contractions had stopped. Part of me functioned as an observer of the scene as if I had floated to the ceiling and looked down at a small, dark-haired woman on a stretcher. She pulled the blankets up to her chin, extended her arm out from under the blanket for a blood pressure check, answered questions.

That was when I unconsciously began to grade each of the staff who spoke to me. I felt like an undercover agent hired to monitor the hospital's quality of care. The nurse who took my history was perfunctory. No kind words, no warmth. I gave her a *C*. I felt sad for all of the patients she had admitted before and would admit after me. She didn't understand how much a soft look, a sympathetic word, or a brief touch on the shoulder would have meant to me. It didn't have to be much, but this nurse wanted "just the facts, ma'am," as if she'd done this admission a hundred times and would do it a hundred more. I might have found some comfort in her matter-of-fact approach. But to me something unexpected was happening, and I needed just a little acknowledgement of that. To her I was an admission at the change of shift: "Thirty-one-year-old nurse in premature labor at twenty-five-weeks gestation, transferred from the Franklin Medical Center in Greenfield. Five feet, four inches tall. One hundred twenty-nine pounds." She apparently wanted only to get the essential information, give report, and go home. Maybe she wanted what I wanted: to be sitting on the sofa in front of the football game with her husband. She filled in the blanks on the forms and handed me and the paperwork over to the next shift.

I wished Jeff would come.

I grew up in Enfield, Connecticut, where my parents still lived. While my ambulance raced down the highway, Jeff retrieved Willie from our neighbor, gathered little boy, blanket, and clothes, and packed for a visit with Grandma and Grandpa. Willie and I had just visited them the day before when Jeff was on call. For me, a Saturday at home alone with a toddler, after a week at home alone with a toddler, loomed long and lonely. After breakfast, I had called Mom and Dad and asked if Willie and I could come for an afternoon visit.

"Of course, Honey," my mother said. "We always love to see you."

In less than an hour, Willie and I were packed and out the door. As I drove south and my body was quiet in the driver's seat, I could not ignore how heavy and achy my upper legs felt. The discomfort was unusual, not at all like muscles that are sore after exercise. I couldn't put my finger on what was wrong, but I had to admit I just did not feel well. I forgot about my symptoms when we arrived in Enfield, and we had a pleasant afternoon with Mom and Dad, who doted on their grandson and on me. But on the way home I drove with one hand on the steering wheel and rubbed my thighs and low back with the other. I wondered if I might be coming down with the flu.

Just as I was being wheeled away to have an ultrasound, Jeff appeared beside the stretcher. He was a little breathless, and he looked frazzled.

"You look as if you've been running," I said to him.

"You gave me directions to the wrong hospital," he said, but without any heat in his voice.

"I did?" I was surprised. "How did I do that?"

"You told me how to get to Wesson Women's Hospital."

"Aren't we at Wesson Women's Hospital?"

"Yes, but you gave me directions to the old hospital. Wesson Women's is part of Baystate now."

I didn't know that in the ten years since I had worked as a nurse's aide at Wesson Memorial Hospital in Springfield, it had become a part of the Baystate Health System. The old building stood where it always had, but the name of the hospital had moved across town. While I was passing through the admissions process and wondering where Jeff was, he was negotiating his way through an unfamiliar city.

I introduced Jeff to the attending obstetrician, Dr. Von Oeyen. I'd met him just before Jeff arrived. The doctor had earned an *A* thus far: he listened to my story, asked good questions, and, bless him, he did not repeat the pelvic exam.

"First, we need to establish exactly how developed the baby is," he said. By dates I was in my twenty-fifth week of pregnancy, but the dates patients remember are not always accurate. Because the labor symptoms were happening so early in the pregnancy, Dr. Von Oeyen wanted to narrow the margin of uncertainty with an ultrasound.

"We can continue to use terbutaline to stop the contractions," he said, "but we need to figure out why your labor started so early." If there was no clear pathological cause, then the labor could be stopped. I could continue the terbutaline and stay on bed rest until the baby was more developed and less at risk for the problems that come with premature birth. I didn't know what other options we had and didn't really want to know at that moment. I just wanted to be carried along on a wave of confidence by specialists who understood this clinical situation.

The abdominal ultrasound estimated I was twenty-five weeks and five days pregnant. That information would help the doctor calculate how much the baby weighed and what its chances would be at birth. Dr. Von Oeyen said he needed to do an amniocentesis to give us the final piece of the puzzle.

An orderly wheeled me into the room where the amniocentesis would be performed. People moved in and out setting up instruments, and rather than being nervous about the procedure itself, I was distracted by a young man in scrubs who seemed to be getting ready to work. His hair was dark, wavy, without a sign of gray, and his face was smooth as if shaving were still just a weekly event for him. He looked to be about twenty.

"Gosh," I whispered to Jeff, "they are getting younger and younger." My lower jaw chattered uncontrollably again. "Do you think this guy is going to do the amnio?"

Jeff bent down to answer me. "I don't think so," he said quietly, his eyes following the subject of our conversation, sizing him up. "He must be a student."

Jeff was right, because Von Oeyen walked in soon after, an air of competence swirling around him, upbeat in spite of being snatched from a Sunday dinner with friends. Recognizing that students have to learn sometime and on somebody, I still breathed easier when the veteran MD snapped on a pair of sterile gloves and turned to pick up the needle and syringe.

Von Oeyen told me he could anesthetize the skin, but then I would feel the burn of the needle and anesthesia instead of the burn of the needle for the amniocentesis itself. I decided to skip local anesthesia even though I had seen the amniocentesis needle where it lay, impressively long and menacing on its sterile field. I felt it pierce the skin of my protruding belly. It sent a burning pain like a streak of lightning through layers of muscle and my uterine wall. I sucked air in and squeezed Jeff's hand. He squeezed back as he glanced from Von Oeyen's hands to the screen above. The doctor worked quickly. Keeping an eye on moving gray shadows on an overhead monitor, he positioned the tip of the needle where he wanted it and then pulled back on the plunger of the large, transparent syringe. He moved with economy, and before I even had a chance to hope the procedure would be over soon, he pulled the needle out and applied pressure to my skin. I let my breath out and forced my muscles to relax. My lower back returned to the table.

The doctor detached the syringe from the needle and handed it to the student. The young man, excited about the procedure he had just witnessed—maybe his first?—held the syringe up to the light in what he assumed to be a professional stance and declared, "Looks pretty clear," and then walked out of the room with the sample.

When everyone left and we were alone in the room, I turned to find Jeff's eyes.

"It didn't look clear to me."

He shook his head and said, "No." He stroked my hair absent-mindedly. "When you started to chill on the way to the ambulance, I wondered if you had an infection."

The cloudy fluid verified his suspicion. Normal amniotic fluid is as clear and colorless as water. It surrounds the fetus and functions as a protective bath. The fluid should not have white cells in it. The cloudiness I could see from across the room probably came from white blood cells hanging suspended in the fluid. The white cells pointed to infection as the probable cause of my early labor.

The picture was beginning to focus. Twelve days earlier, on New Year's Day, I spent a lazy hour on the sofa while Willie drove trucks over the highway that led from my right arm and over my belly to arrive at the palm of my left hand. Reclining in the Cleopatra position, I was able to prolong the languid pace of the holiday morning. Really, though, I needed to start getting ready for a family party. It was my father's fifty-eighth birthday. I was mentally reviewing food preparations and calculating the time I had with a two-hour drive ahead of us when I suddenly felt as if I had started my period. I forced myself off the sofa and walked to the bathroom where I saw something similar to the mucous plug usually released at the beginning of labor. Even though I knew this was unusual at such an early time in pregnancy, I felt no other symptoms.

For whatever complicated reasons, I shrugged off this unusual sign, and I did not call my doctor. I had been living with Jeff and his schedule for years. When he was on call the phone rang constantly. It rang on nights, weekends, and holidays. Most were appropriate calls from sick and worried patients, but too many were for problems that could easily have waited for office hours. Patients seemed to think Jeff was sitting by his phone, waiting for it to ring. I didn't want to be one of those people, and I could not make myself call my obstetrician on New Year's morning. I didn't call the next day, either, because nothing unusual happened after that one event. Over the next two weeks, I went on to develop achy legs and fatigue, but I didn't connect the dots. The symptoms were so subtle I never even told Jeff about them.

Twenty minutes after the amniocentesis, Dr. Von Oeyen joined Jeff and me in a holding room. He pulled up a chair and created a triangular formation as if we were a team huddling together to make a game plan like the football players we'd seen earlier that afternoon. He was the quarterback calling the plays.

"It looks as if you have chorioamnionitis," the doctor said, using a big word whose components I should have been able to figure out as a nurse but could not dissect as a patient. Jeff looked as if he understood but Von Oeyen must have noticed my blank look and continued. "That means infection. Inflammation of the membranes that line the uterine wall."

We were silent, waiting.

"We can't stop the labor if you have an infection," Von Oeyen said. "To do that would be like holding an abscess inside your abdomen. It would be dangerous to you and fatal to the baby."

I don't remember when or how he told us: the baby has to be delivered. I don't remember hearing the words, but it must have been Dr. Von Oeyen who said them.

I was not even two-thirds of the way through my pregnancy.

By the time our conversation with the obstetrician finished it was nearly 8:30 p.m. The lights in the room glowed in a warm way that felt familiar. I had always liked working the evening shift at the hospital. After the bustle of distributing six o'clock medications and getting patients and staff through the confusion of supper, the attending physicians would go home, and harried interns would finally quit writing orders. The floor's activity would settle down to quiet conversations, backrubs, and preparations for bed and the next day's procedures. The late part of the evening shift was more homey than clinical unless the phone rang to signal a new patient coming to the floor. By definition, that person would usually be ill and in need of special attention. On the evening of January 12, I took some comfort from the familiar quiet of the shift. Still, I was the new admission, somebody's problem patient.

The situation seemed increasingly unreal to me as if I were in a car accident with no physical pain. Once, I had had such an experience. I had been one of four nursing students on the way to a psychiatric hospital at eight o'clock on a February morning. One minute we were doing wacky imitations of our professors, and the next we were swirling around and around in a car whose wheels no longer touched the slick surface of the road. There was no pain as we spun. That is how the evening in the obstetrics unit at Baystate felt. Like an emergency without sirens. A 911 call without sound.

Jeff and I had a moment alone while we waited for the anesthesiologist. He took my hand and looked directly at me.

"We need to tell them we don't want any extraordinary measures."
His words were quiet. He meant: no resuscitation if the baby didn't
breathe. No respirator.

I looked at him, and a feeling of sadness washed over me. "Do you
think we have a choice?"

When I worked in pediatric intensive care, I would occasionally float
to the neonatal unit if they needed help. At that time, which was seven
years prior to the night Jeff and I found ourselves at Baystate, NICUs
were saving babies who weighed around two pounds. I understood what
Jeff meant about extraordinary measures. All day he'd been thinking we
were about to lose a pregnancy, not that we were soon to deliver a baby.
But we were in a tertiary care center where every technology for keeping
a premature baby alive was available. Neonatologists and intensive care
nurses specialized in clinical situations precisely like ours. There was no
way they would allow a fully formed, almost twenty-six-week-old fetus
to expire just because the parents were experienced enough to know the
risks of keeping it alive or because we thought the baby would suffer or
for any other reason we might feel was justified.

We knew the chance of it emerging as a normal and healthy baby
was slim. We knew the potential complications: loss of vision from
high oxygen levels, loss of hearing from antibiotics, brain damage or
paralysis from episodes of bleeding within the microscopic vessels of
the still-developing brain. The medical service would use every possible
technology at its disposal to keep this baby alive, and if there were some
illusion that we had a choice in the matter, it was exactly that: an illusion.

I don't think of Jeff as naïve, but I was struck with the innocence
implied in his statement about no extraordinary measures. In his work
as a nephrologist, Jeff takes care of patients whose kidneys have failed
and who require dialysis. Every time a patient shows up for a dialysis
treatment, he or she chooses life for another day. Sometimes patients
decide that a life with so many limitations is too hard, and Jeff helps
patients negotiate that path. He arranges conversations with spiritual
advisors and consults the primary care doctor and family members who
might not want to let go. Patients who are very ill or have many complications often decide not to be resuscitated if their hearts or breathing
should stop. Jeff is used to helping patients and families make choices
about life and death. On that January night, however, he was a husband
and a father as well as a doctor, and he was in unknown territory.

The anesthesiologist entered the room with a grave and earnest manner I appreciated. He pulled up a chair and sat near us in a way that felt sympathetic and approachable. He explained what would happen next and received an *A* for his effort. As he spoke, it became clear he was expecting to attend us through a vaginal delivery. Willie's birth had been by Caesarean section some twenty-six hours after my membranes ruptured because my cervix wouldn't dilate fully. Though it was becoming acceptable in the obstetrical world to attempt vaginal deliveries after C-sections, the idea did not appeal to me. My plan for this pregnancy had been to skip the labor pains and have another Caesarean section. There had not been enough time between pregnancies for me to forget Willie's delivery. To end up in the operating room after enduring around-the-clock contractions was a process I was not anxious to repeat. Of course the situation was different now. I was not delivering an eight-pound baby. I was about to deliver a little creature who might just slip out when I wasn't looking.

My mind jumped ahead. Part of what makes the cervix dilate during labor is the rhythmic pushing of the full-term baby's big round head on the cervix. That pushing—under the strength of the repeated and sustained contractions of the uterine muscle—is what gradually thins and opens the cervical os, much as a chef works a ball of dough into a thin pizza crust. He kneads and pushes the dough over and over against its natural elasticity, against its urge to go back to the tight ball it once was. Pushed and rolled and stretched over time, the ball of dough becomes a thin crust. Knowing the effort it would take even a full term baby to thin the cervix, I visualized the tiny being inside of me trying to do the same thing without the size or stamina of a nine-month-old fetus. How traumatic the process would be for the baby. Going through labor would require that the baby withstand enormous pressure on what must be a very small head, a fragile neck, and vulnerable spinal cord. I thought it impossible for a baby of this size to endure and survive a vaginal delivery.

"I thought I was having a C-section," I said to Jeff and looked to him for validation. His face looked blank. I am not sure we had even discussed it. We were still so far away from the due date, at least three months. I'd just assumed Jeff would agree with my choice.

I looked back at the doctor.

"Can't we do a C-section?" I asked him hopefully. I explained I'd had a Caesarean section with Willie. Though surgery was the riskier choice for me, I knew that because I'd had a C-section with Willie, it was possible they would consider surgery for this delivery. I understood the doctor's unspoken thoughts: the primary goal of the obstetrician and the anesthesiologist was to assure the mother's survival first. The baby, threatened and unlikely to survive the struggles of such an early birth, would be the second priority.

The anesthesiologist responded with raised eyebrows but an alert interest in my question. I couldn't shake the vision of the baby's tiny neck.

"Isn't there more risk to the baby by putting it through labor?" I asked. The baby was still an "it." We didn't know the sex and hadn't asked after the ultrasound. Asking about the gender of this baby seemed frivolous.

"Yes, there is," he admitted.

"Well, then, why can't we do a section if that was my original plan anyway?"

He hesitated before answering. "There is more risk to you if we do surgery with an infection going on." A fact, but I brushed it away. I could see my own medical profile: a young woman in excellent health, no allergies.

"There are plenty of antibiotics for me," I told the doctor. There was no doubt in my mind that I would recover from the surgery. "I'll do fine." I looked at Jeff for confirmation. "If we are really going to save this baby—" a notion I was just getting used to "—then we should give it all the chances we can." As I heard myself speaking, I was half-aware that a switch had flipped in my mind and maybe even in my heart. At that moment, instead of feeling like the helpless victim of a pregnancy gone wrong, I became a mother trying to save her child. Surgery seemed better for the baby and me. I could not imagine going through hours of labor, chilled, trembling, and feeling as if I had the flu, not knowing when it was going to end. Neither could I imagine a tiny undeveloped baby, not at all ready to be in the world, enduring hours of stress, pushing through an unripe cervix, and surviving the ordeal. Surgery would be better for both of us. Us. My baby and me.

I pushed aside the things I knew about premature babies for the moment: respiratory distress syndrome, necrotizing enterocolitis, blindness, brain damage. There wasn't room for ambivalence. I could only think into the next few hours, and apparently Jeff and I were about to have a baby. If that was the plan, then we had to give him or her the best possible chance for survival.

The anesthesiologist agreed to the idea of surgery, and Jeff supported my choice. Apparently there was no difficulty persuading Dr.

Von Oeyen to go the surgical route. From a practical perspective, it was quicker to whisk me into the operating room on this Sunday evening and do a thirty-minute procedure than it would be to sit through the night with a high-risk labor that might or might not progress. It was clear which choice would work in the baby's favor.

I watched as a nurse took Jeff by the arm and led him away to prepare to be in the operating room with me. Usually a birthing partner has to go to special prenatal classes in order to attend a C-section, but because he was a physician, Jeff was allowed to come with me to the operating room.

Given the options, I chose to have spinal anesthesia. Though I could have been put under general sedation, my head and heart wanted to be there for every minute of the birth. I needed to see what happened to the baby from the first breath. From the first cry, if the baby cried at all. If the baby did not survive, I did not want to wake up to the news. Still, I was fairly certain that the baby would not die at birth. The neonatal team and its equipment would make it difficult for a baby, even a premature one, to die. I had to see for myself whether the birth was the beginning or the end of the story.

A nurse rolled my stretcher into the operating room, a cold and white space gleaming with sterility. After the awkward transfer from stretcher to operating table, I turned onto my right side. The nurse slipped her hands under my hips and adjusted my body in a position for spinal anesthesia. Though I wanted to be awake for the surgery, I was still nervous about trusting someone to stick a needle into my spine. I couldn't help but remember stories of spinals gone bad. I kept thinking, I hope this guy knows what he's doing. I want to be able to walk when I get out of here.

As I lay on my side with a nurse supporting me in my best effort at a fetal position, I felt cold swabbing on my lower back. I smelled Betadine solution. Then, through the neutralized touch of a gloved hand, I could feel the anesthesiologist palpating the ladder of bones in my lower back. He was quick and confident, and I knew he had experience in his fingertips. A prick of the needle anesthetized my skin, and after a few moments there was more pressure on my low back and then a buzz that zoomed down my legs. Before I had time to say, "I have this weird feeling in my legs," the anesthesiologist was saying to me, "It's normal to feel a buzzing sensation in your legs." He continued to earn his *A*. Within minutes, I was straightened out and lying on my back again. Numbness started first at my feet, then rose to my knees, my thighs, and over the expanse of my belly.

As the staff prepared for surgery, the operating room assumed a solemn and ceremonious air. I could see shining eyes, intense with the energy of the moment, oases of warmth above the blue masks. The scrub nurse moved around the room, her choreography worked out and practiced with other patients who had preceded me and the birthing of other babies before mine. I heard orders murmured from behind one of the masks. Muffled voices asked and answered questions in warped time, a seventy-eight record playing on thirty-three speed. A face came down to mine and blocked the light that glowed from behind his head like a halo. The voice behind the mask belonged to the anesthesiologist, and he asked what I felt, "Here?" Poking me with something, I supposed. "Here?" I felt nothing.

A mirror hung from the ceiling and was positioned so Jeff could watch the surgery. The room became almost festive then, everyone charged and excited once they had something to do. It was odd to realize my lower parts were being pushed and then manipulated into position as the nurse told me she was swabbing my abdomen with something like a big paintbrush. I could feel my body moving but the motion wasn't under my control. The lower half of me felt as if it belonged to someone else. It tingled a bit like a fat, numb lip after dental work. One of the blue-clad figures opened a drape and set up a tent, separating the small part of me that felt alive from the larger part of me I could no longer feel. Then the fat numbness began to move upward, extending as high as my breasts. Is it normal to be numb all the way to my chest? I wondered but couldn't make my mouth work to ask. I thought the anesthesia was supposed to go down to my feet, not up to my chest. I started to feel panicky. Can it affect my lungs? Will I stop breathing? How long will it take them to figure out they gave me too much medication and I am not breathing? But my chest continued to move air in and out. I paid attention to every breath. I worried if I didn't, the breathing might stop.

A nurse gave Jeff specific instructions about where to sit. He was on a stool up with the live part of me. He stroked my hair, touched my shoulder, rubbed my arm. He said little. His eyes stared at a point beyond the tent.

Finally Dr. Von Oeyen faced the table. I saw him hold his gloved hands suspended in the air. The nurse smacked a scalpel into the doctor's palm, and he said "Ready? Here we go." I knew someone would start a timer. From the moment the scalpel pierced through the skin of my abdomen, they had a small window of time to deliver the baby safely. The baby needed to have a source of oxygen through the entire surgery. In an instant, he or she would make a dramatic transition from getting oxygen via the umbilical cord to breathing air into newly expanding lungs.

The upper, conscious part of me felt insignificant to the unfolding drama. I was just the vehicle. The action moved to a place at the other end of my body at the far end of the table. Jeff's hand rested on my shoulder, but his eyes had refocused and were riveted on the mirror. Even the anesthesiologist, whose job was to monitor my vital signs, was caught up in the suspense. In that long minute, blue-gowned shoulders and surgical caps moved in and out of my view beyond the drape as I felt my body being pushed in a quiet violence. Then I heard it—the tiniest cry, just one half-hearted mew like a cat would make if it wanted breakfast but knew it was not really time. A subdued male voice said, "You have a girl."

The words announcing that my pregnancy was now a baby girl, a being who two days before had been no more than a stretching of my waistline and some flutters under my ribs, dropped like a stone into the still waters of a lake. I knew, with her cry, that my baby had breathed immediately. She would not need to be resuscitated, and her first breath was nothing less than a miracle. But that was all I knew. A team of backs and shoulders from a different group, who wore green, converged somewhere beyond and to the left of my feet. The action moved from my body to the baby's. The energy surge that had come into the operating suite with the surgery and the inkling of hope I felt when I heard my baby cry swirled away, slowly at first, then in a quickening vortex, like the bath water Willie would watch intently as it swept the remnants of his day down the drain.

SUNDAY, CONTINUED:
THE NIGHT SHIFT

In December of 1984 when we celebrated our first Massachusetts Christmas, we sent holiday cards from our new home to our old friends back in Washington. We included a photograph of five-month-old Willie, who'd been a newborn when we packed up our red station wagon and two golden retrievers and left the Northwest. We also sent cards to our family doctor and the anesthesiologist who had attended Willie's birth. A few weeks after that Christmas, I opened a letter that was postmarked "Wenatchee, WA." I was surprised to see it was from the anesthesiologist, of all people, dated January 1, 1985. He wrote: "Please accept my humble gratitude for your kind Christmas note. Your delivery was one of the more memorable ones to me for the obvious great love which exists between the two of you. It was touching to me and I was pleased to have had the opportunity to share it with you. And from the picture it is obvious that all three of you are doing well."

During that labor with Willie, Jeff had been attentive for twenty-six hours, supporting me through contractions, helping me breathe with the pains. Though he had resisted attending Lamaze classes, he had come through as an ideal labor partner, and he was vigilant during Willie's birth. After they said, "It's a boy!" and we both cried, hugged, and wiped away our tears with the sleeve of my hospital gown, he squeezed my shoulder and said, "I have to go see my son." He moved down to the warmer to join our family doctor, and after a nurse weighed and measured the still-unnamed little boy, Jeff held our baby for the first time.

None of the joy that had been a part of Willie's birth entered the operating room on the Sunday evening when our second child—our daughter—was delivered. Though this was not an emergency C-section, there was enough urgency in the situation to keep the mood solemn.

We heard the baby's cry after eleven o'clock at the end of a day that could not possibly have started with a routine pancake breakfast. I lay on the operating table and felt empty, then confused, then angry, with no one to blame and no way to explain why it had all gone wrong. "You have a girl" hit me like a slap, left my cheek burning with the sting of it. This was not the scene I'd visualized for this baby. I was looking for a seven-and-a-half-pound little girl who was to have been born in April when daffodils would be blooming in my yard. Instead, we were in the deepest part of winter. She met fluorescent white light in a room that smelled of antiseptics and heard the murmur of subdued voices mixed with the clang of surgical instruments. I couldn't see anything of her through the wall of blue and green scrubs. I never had even a glimpse of her that night.

Though she breathed on her own right away, the baby was intubated soon after her first breath because, at her size, she would not have enough energy to breathe independently for any length of time. I knew what was happening. A neonatologist inserted an endotracheal tube into her mouth where the tip moved past her vocal chords and into the trachea. The other end attached to tubing that led to a ventilator, not a big boxy machine like the ones for adults, but a much smaller piece of equipment capable of puffing breaths of air titrated for a miniature human being. Pushing oxygenated air into her lungs, the machine breathed for her.

"Sarah?" I heard myself say. I looked at Jeff for confirmation, and looking in her direction, he nodded, not meeting my eyes. Within minutes the team whisked the baby out of the operating room to whatever awaited her. We hadn't talked about names yet, but Sarah Katherine was the name we had been sure of when Willie was born if he had been born a she. Without putting the thought into words, I felt it would have been a breach of faith to call her something different from the name we had chosen before. Still, part of me wondered if we should use it on a baby who might not live long enough to know her name.

After the neonatology team took the baby away, the surgical team still needed to finish the job of putting me back together. The atmosphere in the room seemed to deflate. Quiet routine resumed. Then, as I lay there, numb in my heart as well as my body, I noticed the beginning of the same sensation I had experienced after Willie's delivery. It was the sense of shivering without being cold. Earlier in the evening I had explained to the anesthesiologist that during Willie's delivery I had developed an uncontrollable shaking reaction, like a chill, though I hadn't felt cold.

"The shaking is a common response to spinal anesthesia," he said. "If it happens this time, I'll give you something to stop it."

My arms began to tremble, and then I found my jaw, neck, arm, and chest muscles shaking uncontrollably. I wondered if this was an anxiety attack, but I knew what I was feeling was not anxiety. I felt sad. Perhaps this shaking was from fever, a chill coming on. Whatever the cause, I began to feel afraid. It felt as if all of the muscles not paralyzed by the anesthesia were in a trembling spasm. My teeth chattered as if someone had thrown open the windows of the surgical suite to the cold January night. The anesthesiologist noticed the reaction—it was from the medication, he assured me—and from the corner of my eye I could see his gloved hands draw fluid from a bottle into a syringe. He inserted the needle into the rubber IV port and slowly moved his thumb on the plunger, adding one invisible liquid to the other. Almost immediately, miraculously, the spasms ceased. I felt my body sink down again onto the surgical table, and my arms, chest, and face succumbed to heaviness. I closed my eyes with relief.

Jeff kissed my forehead and whispered a goodbye and "I love you" into my ear. He might as well leave. He couldn't see the baby, and as far as he could tell I was sedated. I heard him say he was going to my parents' house for the night.

I tried to say good-bye to him, but my mouth wouldn't work. My eyes wouldn't open either. I couldn't move my hand to hold onto him. What was going on? The fear I'd been trying to suppress started to grow.

I could hear murmured conversation and lay still, trying not to panic. A few minutes after Jeff departed, I noticed a feeling in my abdomen. What was it? The sensation of pushing and pulling I had been aware of earlier, when I first received the spinal anesthesia, was coming back. It was a blurry discomfort at first, but then it grew, all too quickly, into a focused pain, building in volume, filling my consciousness. Suddenly the pain was surrounding me in a black swirl as huge and as evil as the bad guy in the *Sleeping Beauty* video that Willie liked to watch over and over again.

The anesthesia was wearing off. I wanted to say the words, but once again my mouth, my entire face, would not work. My eyes would not open. The IV medication had taken effect and quieted the spasms in my muscles, but the additional effect was that I couldn't move at all. The medication stopped the trembling but left me unable to move my hands, my arms, or my mouth. After the injection, I could feel I was breathing on my own but had no control over any part of my body, and from the depths of a brain that was all too awake, I wanted to scream. I felt as if I were in a nightmare as I tried to run with legs that refused to move, tried to cry out with a hand over my mouth, but in this un-dream I experienced no moment of sitting upright in the bed, sweating. I could not move out of the nightmare. The mass of pain engulfed and surrounded me, and all of my nerve endings were electrified.

I was alone. Jeff didn't know about the pain. He didn't know that I was pleading, come back! I can feel this! I can feel all of it! I couldn't tell him, and he couldn't rescue me.

In real time, I wonder how long the closure of the incision really took. In my drugged blur, I lay in another dimension where time was not measured by hands on a clock. I could hear Von Oeyen talking a resident through the stapling. As far as they could see, their patient rested comfortably. She was quiet and cooperative. They had no idea I was aware of every fiber in my skin and muscle wall and uterus that had been severed by the scalpel. The snap of the staple gun interrupted the quiet of the room as the operating team bent over their work, and though they could see under the skin, between the muscles, and through the blood vessels and nerves of my pelvis, they remained oblivious to my pain.

I knew I had reached the recovery room when I felt the temperature around me drop as if I had been rolled into a refrigerator. My stretcher was lined up with a bed. Hands rolled the sheet that was underneath my shoulders, my back, my now-tingling legs. Without any help from me, they moved my body "One, two, three!" onto yet another bed. I still could not form words with my mouth and couldn't tell anyone that my abdomen felt as if it had been hit by a grenade. After positioning my limbs and arranging the blankets over me, the recovery room nurse gave me an injection of Demerol, not because I had been able to ask but because that was what the doctor ordered after surgery. As nurses, we work on "staying ahead" of pain by medicating a patient before the pain gets intense. But they were too late with this pain—they were way behind and it was out of control. The injection was a benevolent thought but laughable in its effect, like tilting a watering can onto a forest fire. It did nothing to ease the pain.

I knew there were at least two males in the recovery room. I could hear quiet conversation somewhere beyond my limited vision. But the IV medicine the anesthesiologist had given me was still working, and I could not yet speak. The nurse's post-op note probably read, "Thirty-one-year-old female admitted to RR post C-section for premature labor secondary to chorioamnionitis. No fever. Vital signs stable. Appears comfortable." I could barely see from under heavy eyelids as the blue scrubs moved out of the room, and I tried to make the words: so much pain. But the doctors looked me over and, satisfied with what they saw, they walked out of the room.

When the paralysis gradually wore off and my arm did what I told it to do, I pointed at the nurse with my index finger. She saw me and came to my bedside. Struggling to make my mouth and tongue work, I tried to tell her about the pain.

"You've already had a shot of Demerol," she said, not unkindly, but as if I should know better than to ask for more.

"I know," I said to her. I tried in a slurry way to explain about the anesthesia, how it had worn off during the surgery and the pain was huge, bigger than the room we were in, but she looked at me with suspicion. I knew she did not believe I should have this pain. She had followed the post-op orders. She had given me the shot of Demerol upon my arrival in the recovery room. As I lay there in the bright white of a room that felt as cold and unsympathetic as a meat locker, I asked forgiveness from every patient whom I had ever made wait for pain medication, for all the times the light had been on over someone's door and I had run to do something else first or had rolled my eyes and looked at my watch "knowing" it was too soon for the patient's codeine or Demerol or morphine. On that night, I was not the nurse with the key to the narcotics cabinet. I was the patient, and the pain continued to fill and surround my abdomen and back, radiating to every nerve.

Later, when I looked at the scar across my lower abdomen, I wondered that a six-inch incision could hurt so much. But, of course, the cut went deeper than what I could see. The surgeon had to slice through abdominal muscles, through the uterus, and then he manipulated and disrupted those muscles and organs in ways they are never meant to be handled. The sensation originated as single notes in the severed nerves from each of those places but then radiated from the core of my body into a full crescendo of pain. Finally, when the clock indicated that the correct interval had passed, the nurse gave me a second injection of Demerol. It took some time for the medication to quiet the agony that had been with me for hours, but I eventually fell into a semi-conscious doze.

Sometime after three that morning my vital signs were stable. The gurney reappeared.

"You'll be leaving us now," the nurse said. "You are being transferred to the high-risk obstetrics floor." More sheet-pulling and log-rolling, and then the nurse said, "Good luck, Dear," as the ceiling began to move above me once again.

The halls of the hospital were quiet though the lights in the halls blazed as if it were midday. Hospital scenes rolled by in a haze as we passed through the building and up elevators to the fifth floor. The squeaky wheels of the gurney and the mechanics of the elevator doors seemed a noisy insult in the sleeping building.

In contrast to the bright elevator and hallways, the lights on the obstetrical floor glowed softly as I rolled down the hall, and the patient rooms were dark. Finally we stopped and turned into a room.

Oh . . . oh . . . careful . . . my belly, I thought as once again I was turned and rolled and hoisted from the gurney to a new bed with a confusion of arm-board, IV bag, tubing, and sheets to be disentangled. Then I was alone in the quiet of a four-bed room, the other women trying to sleep through a middle-of-the-night admission. Feeling unsettled in yet another new place—how many beds had I lain in over the last sixteen hours?—I didn't know what to expect from the night. Continuing pain, for sure. Sleep, I hoped, though that seemed unlikely.

I wondered what was happening to the baby. She was just down the hall, but that was an impossible distance from me. We hadn't even been properly introduced.

After the transport people left, someone came into the room and moved silently around my bed—a nurse, I could finally see when she came into my range of vision—organizing my body and the post-operative equipment. I sensed rather than saw her check the drip of the IV. I opened my mouth for a thermometer. She took my blood pressure, leaving the cuff on my arm. She lifted the sheet and my gown and looked at my dressing, checking for any visible drainage, I knew. The sheets smelled industrially clean and felt rough and cold. She moved to the end of the bed to loosen the corners from their military tuck so that I could wiggle my toes. How did she know to do that, I wondered. She took the thermometer from my mouth, and then she offered a back massage.

I had never worked on a surgical floor. I wouldn't have thought to give a backrub after surgery, but of course it made sense. I had been immobile for hours, unable to shift my legs or change the pressure on my buttocks. My muscles were stiff. Even my skin was sore. Though I didn't think it was possible to change my position in my miserable state, the nurse turned me on my side with gentle dexterity. She lifted one of my legs and crossed it over the other, then pulled and adjusted my weight onto one hip. When she was satisfied with the position of the lower half of my body, she carefully moved my shoulders into alignment with the rest of me.

"Everyone else is sleeping," the nurse said as she worked. "You have me all to yourself." She turned the full beam of her attention on me.

The night moved forward in slow motion. "Tell me about your baby." The voice behind me asked questions while her fingers moved over my skin and muscles, the long, smooth strokes of her hands absorbing my sadness and easing the hurt. When I told her a bumpy version of what had happened that day and evening, then about the surgery and the anesthesia that didn't last, she walked out of the room and returned as quickly with another injection for the pain. She let the medicine and the massage do their work. After some minutes of silence between us, she told me that her son, in his early twenties, had died unexpectedly in an accident the year before.

Although it is easy to feel cut off when a listener interjects her own story, this nurse knew how to listen and when to share. In that quiet, dark hour before the day began, before my life would take off from a new starting point, she talked gently about her son. Hearing her words helped me regain some perspective about my daughter. She didn't say the words, but I heard them: I have great sympathy for you, but you are not the only mother to have experienced loss. You may not believe it tonight, but you will survive. She reframed the picture for me, and I hung onto a fuzzy memory of her words in the following days as I struggled with a new concept of family.

I never saw the nurse's face in the subdued light. To this day, I visualize her surrounded by a Florence Nightingale kind of glow. Her attention to my body and then my heart has since caused me to search my memory, wondering . . . hoping . . . that in my years as a nurse, I might possibly have given such a gift to a patient in a time of pain or fear or need. The nurse who admitted me to the fifth floor on the night of Sarah's birth had found her calling. She was like an angel, placed in the hospital to do a good deed for a patient who happened to lie in a bed along the path on which she, the nurse, was destined to walk that night. I do not remember the nurse's name, and I never saw her after that shift ended.

January nights are long. I don't know how much time the nurse spent with me, but it was enough to smooth out the wrinkles left from that long day. Under the influence of the Demerol injection and the nurse's sure hands and comforting words, I fell into a dreamless sleep.

TAKING CARE OF BUSINESS

Jeff had few phone calls to make the night Sarah was born. He called his parents, of course, but we didn't have many local friends. We'd been residents of Massachusetts for only a year and a half, and everyone knows it takes Yankees a while to warm up to newcomers. Soon after we arrived in Gill, Jeff plunged into his new job as the director of the dialysis unit at the hospital in Greenfield, and he was welcomed there and into the community at large with open arms and a busy schedule. He had also joined an internal medicine practice with six other physicians, so his life instantly became a series of long workdays followed by nights and weekends on call.

I, on the other hand, stayed home. Though I was ready and happy to be a mother, many of my friends and colleagues lived out west. They were the people who had known me as the person I'd been before becoming a mother. When I left those people, it seemed that I left a big part of myself as well.

On the positive side, moving to Massachusetts did place me within a two-hour drive of my parents and my sister Lorie, but we weren't physically close enough to share the humdrum of the average day. Jeff and I had met in New Haven, so we knew some people there, but that is also a two-hour drive from Gill. Jeff had a college friend living in a town not far from Baystate, but we had seen him and his wife only a few times since we moved back east. The weeks turned into months of feeling a little disoriented even in my own home where I tried to figure out how my life should be with a new baby in a new town and a "hold" button flashing on my professional life.

On Tuesday and Thursday mornings, Willie and I attended a swim-and-gym class at the Greenfield YMCA. We both screeched and shivered through the swim part. After we had done the requisite penance in the pool, the class moved to the gym. I chatted with other mothers while the children swarmed at our legs. Thus far they had been "Y only" friends.

How to make friends? I was no longer a student or a working nurse, no longer traveling and doing temporary stints of nursing as I had for a few years. When we lived in Salt Lake City and I was a graduate student at the University of Utah, the tightly-knit Mormon community left the city's non-Mormon residents to gravitate towards one another, and casual acquaintances quickly turned into friends who were ready to meet for a quick and cheap dinner. Friendships seemed to spring forth into something immediately nourishing, like an instant breakfast powder that comes from a package—just add the missing element. First it was beer and a pizza. Then we expanded to afternoons on the ski slopes, hikes up canyon trails, or, in Jeff's case, hours spent with a squash racquet in hand.

Friendships did not develop as readily in rural New England. I needed to go to work, just a little, to dip my toe in professional waters and to be assured of conversation a few times each week with someone other than Jeff and Willie. As 1985 drew to a close, I had two fill-in-the-gap part-time jobs, but none of my co-workers had progressed to the status of after-work friends. We all were juggling little kids and baskets of laundry and husbands along with our jobs. I looked forward to seeing my colleagues on the days I worked.

I worked weekends at the walk-in clinic at UMass, and Thursday afternoons at the family planning clinic across the street from the Green-field hospital. By January of 1986, three of the family planning staff—Jean the RN, Sarah the exam room assistant, and I—were noticeably pregnant. Sarah was really a photographer trying to stay away from developing chemicals during her pregnancy, and her due date was in January. Jean was due in March, and I, in April. One afternoon, I turned sideways in order to squeeze past Jean in the narrow hallway of the clinic. We had a big laugh about how we, the staff, were the poster girls for what our afternoon roster of clients should not look like if we were successful at our work.

On the evening of January 12, in the lull between when the doctors left us and I was wheeled off to surgery, Jeff and I had found a quiet moment to talk about the week ahead. As I lay on the bed in the hospital room and Jeff and I made plans for a week we couldn't even begin to visualize, I once again found myself observing the scene from above. My thinking brain and my feelings seemed to be functioning independently of one another, divided down the middle by an objective, rational line. While my emotions were caught up in the unfolding events, the cognitive portion of my mind was still able to anticipate the mundane requirements of daily existence: the dog to care for, the work obligations I wouldn't be available to fulfill, and the appointments that would have to be changed. The details seemed clear enough, but very small, as if I were looking at the days ahead through the wrong end of binoculars. I asked Jeff to call family planning and the UMass health center to tell them I would be out of work indefinitely. Somehow I also remembered to ask him to call my colleague Sarah from family planning to let her know I would not be arriving at her house the next morning. She was the closest I had come to having a friend outside of work, and we had planned to meet on Monday, January 13, for a morning of cross-country skiing.

Once I had checked those pieces of business off my mental list, it was as if I started a new chapter in a book. There was nothing gentle about the story after that. I was swept into it as if on a wave bursting through a dam. While I tried to keep my nose above the water's surface on that swirling ride, the ski day I had planned with my new friend, the swim-and-gym class on Tuesday, the dental appointment on Wednesday, and the refrigerator that needed to be restocked, all seemed to belong to a life I could remember but whose wide-eyed innocence I already thought of in the past tense.

MOTHERING BY PROXY

After I returned from that first trip to the NICU the morning after the baby was born, I picked up the phone. It had been very quiet. I hadn't spoken to anyone outside of the hospital yet. Jeff had come by earlier that morning—or had I dreamed that? I wasn't sure.

I called my mother to see how she and Willie were doing. It was the first time we had spoken since our Saturday visit at her house when I had still been pregnant.

"I'm so glad I told you I loved you when you were leaving on Saturday," she said, her voice wobbling. "How is she?"

My mother has many strengths, but her ability to tolerate the things that happen in hospitals is not among them. I could feel her wincing at the other end of the phone as I told her how the baby looked and what little I knew. I told her the doctors weren't projecting much into the future. Not months. Not days. Not even hours.

"Poor little darlin'," was all she could manage.

There wasn't much more to say about the baby, so we moved on in the conversation. "Willie is fine," she said. Then she peppered me with questions.

"When does he nap?" she asked. "Does he like baths these days? Will he let me wash his hair? When does he usually go to bed?" She gathered the information a grandmother needed, and I was certain Willie would have his every wish granted. He had been with Grandma for less than twenty-four hours, and she was already teaching him the words for colors with the magnetic letters she had found at a tag sale.

"He's so smart!" she said as if I needed convincing.

My brain was fuzzing over, and we soon said our goodbyes. With the responsibilities of motherhood out of my hands, I did the only thing I was capable of doing. Ignoring the parade of lab technicians, nurses, doctors, and family members who trooped in and out of the four-bed room, I let the pain medicines take control. I pulled the covers up to my chin, turned gingerly onto one side, and closed my eyes.

After my lunch of tea and Jell-O, a cheerful nurse bounced into my room. I learned that there was, after all, something I could give the baby.

"I'm here to teach you how to express milk for your baby until she can feed on her own," the nurse announced, her voice all exclamation points.

"Breast-feed?" I asked, feeling stupid. What is she talking about? I thought. Has she seen my baby?

"Oh, yes," she assured me. "Mothers often feed their preemies successfully. You just have to pump your breasts four times a day to keep your milk supply going until the baby can nurse. In the meantime I've brought an electric breast pump"—she nodded toward a machine that sat on a stainless steel cart—"and I will give you some little Baggies, so you can store the milk in your freezer."

Then she stopped for a moment, her brow furrowed.

"Are you on any antibiotics?"

"Yes, I am."

"Oh, well," she wavered for a moment and then surged forward, undaunted, "in that case you'll have to discard your milk until you are off the medication. You can start saving it two days after you are finished with the antibiotics."

The woman probably chose to be a La Leche nurse because she liked teaching happy, excited new mothers the wonders of breast-feeding. Those mothers would lie in bed with their babies curled in their arms, and she would help them to adjust pillows and find comfortable positions for nursing. I must have been a disappointment as I stared at the nurse in my drugged, hollow-eyed stupor. She positioned the machine close to the bed and plugged the cord into the wall socket. Then she handed me a white plastic bottle with a funnel-like top. Apparently I was supposed to place the funnel up to my breast. After connecting the suction bottle to the tubing and the tubing to the machine, the nurse gathered her teaching tools and swept out of the room. I was left with a box of empty Baggies in a space that echoed with her misplaced enthusiasm.

In the wake of the nurse's bright energy, I sat behind the curtain she had pulled around my bed for privacy and flipped the toggle switch that turned the machine on. It was obnoxiously loud and a little scary to feel my breast being rhythmically sucked and released, sucked and released in the funnel top of the plastic bottle. The machine whined in a relentless on-off cycle, pulling a meager stream of thin, gray fluid from my breast. I felt an immediate revulsion towards the pump. At first I tried to visualize the good of this colostrum, the first nourishment my body would make for the baby, but I knew I would just be tossing the liquid down the sink. My mind stubbornly went back to memories of sitting on the living room sofa with Willie at my breast. We were a cozy pair from the warm days of July all the way until the wood stove warmed the room that winter. He would lie in my arms, his eyes at half-mast, his hands moving from the folds of his ear to the warmth of my skin as if he were reading Braille. I had stopped nursing him when he was nine months old. Now, just nine months after I'd stopped nursing Willie, I sat in a hospital room with the cold, impersonal grinding of an electric motor, but without a baby to stimulate the tingling of milk that would have willingly flowed through my breasts.

On that first day of pumping I dribbled the same volume of tears as I did breast milk. Then every four hours I did as I had been told, dutifully hiding myself behind the mechanical noise and the curtain. I endured the pumping in order to make what I feared was the only contribution I could to my baby's welfare.

DAY TWO

On Tuesday, when my stomach proved it could tolerate the toast and tea on my breakfast tray, I moved to the regular obstetrics floor. There I was, one patient on a corridor with many women who were pregnant, post-miscarriage, post-partum, whatever. The only requirement was that we be female with some reproductive health problem. The floor was busy, and as one of the less complicated patients there, I felt invisible. Though I was newly post-operative, I didn't need much beyond the IV antibiotics and an occasional look under my surgical dressing. I was in a four-bed room occupied by one other woman, an unmoving hump in the bed directly across from me. Within a short time, another patient was admitted to the room. As soon as she was settled in bed, she picked up the phone and started pushing buttons.

I had been attempting to read, but I couldn't help noticing my new roommate. She looked young, not more than seventeen, I thought, as she warmed to her telephone conversation. When a nurse rolled a bassinet into the room, the girl didn't miss a line of her dialogue and never even glanced sideways at the baby who lay in the portable crib parked next to her bed. I could hear her side of the conversation, and it was not about the baby.

"He said what?" she said into the phone. "Andthenwhatdidhedo? Really?" She laughed. More talk. The nurse in me roiled as I watched the girl ignore the newborn infant who lay swaddled in a blue receiving blanket.

I couldn't watch, and I couldn't not watch. A mild squeaking started from the bassinet and began to work itself into something more insistent until the nurse reappeared and, unable to hide her disapproval of her patient's un-maternal behavior, picked the blue bundle up and handed him to his mother. The teen acknowledged the gesture by wedging the phone between her head and shoulder and taking the baby. She began to jiggle the bundle. She still hadn't looked at her baby. Finally, when the nurse handed the mother a bottle, she hung up the phone and turned her attention to feeding the infant. The girl did not acknowledge the nurse, who said few words to the mother, and there were no kisses for her child. No baby talk. She did not look into his face or touch his hands. Her behavior was so perfunctory that it occurred to me with a stab that this baby might not have been the young woman's first child. When the phone rang again, she got herself situated with phone-to-shoulder and bottle-to-baby, and the conversation picked up where it had been interrupted.

My eyes filled. I didn't mean to cry, but in the brief time I'd spent watching that baby with his mother, I saw the trajectory of his life as clearly as if someone had written his biography and placed it on my bedside table. I reached down to find the electrical controls on the side of my bed and lowered the head. Maybe if I didn't see them, I could ignore what was going on across the way. I lay there hurting, both for my own baby and for the one across the room. I ached to have a whole baby I could hold up in the air at arm's length to just look at, to see her face, her eyes that indefinable new-baby blue. I wanted the things I had luxuriated in with Willie in the hours after his birth: examining the perfectly formed ears that lay flat on the sides of his molded head; marveling over his long, wrinkled fingers; searching through the receiving blanket to find long feet and pearly toes all curled and pink.

How could this mother not see the miracle of her baby?

And then I realized she couldn't see her baby because she was only a child herself. She was an adolescent who mostly wanted to sit by the phone and talk to her friends. She had no idea how to fit a baby into her life.

I looked up at my IV bag and thought that the fluid must be running into my vein and then directly out of my eyes. I could feel a headache developing in the back of my head, and it started to bang, bang, bang with my pulse. I couldn't stop the sound of the young mother's voice, the squeaky fussing of the baby, or the overflow of my tears.

The floor buzzed with activity that morning, and the staff ran in all directions. I felt silly having to ask a nurse or an aide to wheel me to the NICU when they had work to do. I was two floors away from the baby yet unable to go to the unit when I wanted to. I felt imprisoned. All of the protocols I had to work around—calling the unit first to see if I could come, getting transportation, scrubbing my hands for five minutes and dressing in a gown before entering the NICU—made me feel confined and frustrated. But with the drama unfolding across the room, I needed to get out and up the stairs to see my own baby. Sarah. I needed to get used to calling her that.

I swung my legs over the side of the bed to test them. Jeff had brought my robe on the previous evening, so I slipped my free arm into one sleeve and draped the robe's other shoulder over the arm that was connected to the IV. Hanging onto the pole for support, I stood up and straightened slowly. Once I was semi-upright and the horizon seemed to be holding steady, I shuffled out of the room and took a right towards the elevator. Feeling like a prison escapee I looked over my shoulder, worried that someone would come running after me and yell, "Hey Lady! Where do you think you're going?" But no one did. When I reached the end of the hallway, I pushed the UP button on the wall and waited for the elevator.

A nurse had helped me with a shower earlier that morning. At least I had washed off the residue of sweat and surgery, but I had forgotten to ask Jeff to bring my slippers, so the hospital's green scuffs peeked out from under my robe. I'd combed my hair after the shower but hadn't fussed beyond that. I knew my appearance had to be institutional, at best. Visitors in street dress and hospital staff in scrubs pushed to the back of the elevator as I moved slowly into their midst, their eyes darting away from me and my IV pole and the garb that identified me as a patient.

As the elevator began to move, two opposing sensations overtook my body. The firm, white bones of my skeleton seemed to be traveling up with the elevator, while my soft tissues—heart, liver, stomach, stitched-up uterus, and brain—were sinking down as if my blood were draining into the elevator shaft. When the door opened to the fifth floor, I looked at the space between the threshold of the elevator car and the squares of linoleum floor and wondered how I would step from one to the other, how I would negotiate the three black wheels that swiveled at the bottom of my IV pole over what appeared to be an insurmountable moat. I used the pole to support myself, nausea now churning, sweat breaking over my entire skin, and I scuffed each foot, left, right, left, across the hall to the wall opposite the elevator. How dumb, I thought. I am going to faint. I continued moving, but in slow motion. I should lie down on the floor, I reasoned, raise my legs. But where can I? Right here in the middle of the hall? Too public. Too many germs. If I can just make it to that wall. No, I can't move fast enough . . .

The bright fluorescence of the hallway faded, and the black spots floating in front of my eyes coalesced into a blank emptiness. I felt my body sink to the floor.

That afternoon, the nurse for the evening shift introduced herself as she started her rounds. Gayle asked how I was feeling since my declaration of independence and subsequent rescue earlier in the day, and she made me promise to ask for help when I wanted to go to the NICU again. I told her Jeff would be coming in the evening, and I would wait until then to visit the baby. She checked my temperature and pulse and measured the amount of fluid left in the IV with a quick glance. I could see her eye assessing the needs of her other charges in the room even as she measured my blood pressure with the stethoscope. Though I had just started to see her in action, I gave Gayle a quick *A*.

"Could I get some Tylenol?" I asked while I had her beside me. "I have such a headache." I didn't want to complain about the diarrhea from the antibiotics, about the commotion in a four-bed room and the roommate who neglected her perfect baby, about not being able to get upstairs to see my baby when I wanted to, about the headache that pounded like a hammer trying to break my skull open from the inside.

"It must be from all the crying," I said, embarrassed. Gayle looked over at the mountain of tissues piled up in my wastebasket.

"A headache?" She was listening even as she wrote my vital signs on the clipboard she took from its spot at the end of my bed. "You had spinal anesthesia, didn't you?"

"I did," I answered, hearing her question and wondering why I hadn't thought of it myself.

Gayle's nursing antennae had been vibrating in the few moments of what had been a very brief conversation, and she suspected the headache was not from crying but was more likely due to the spinal anesthesia. Usually the tiny hole made by the needle in the lining of the spinal cord seals itself once the needle is removed. Sometimes, though, the pinhole leaks, and when it does, the volume of spinal fluid is reduced and the brain has less padding where it sits inside the hard cranium. Without enough cushioning, the brain sort of rattles around and then comes the headache. Once the hole seals and the fluid rebuilds itself, the pain goes away, but that can take weeks. I had a vision of my future self running the vacuum cleaner in my living room, my head pounding.

"I'll call anesthesia," she said.

In less than an hour an anesthesia resident was at my bedside asking questions about the headache. His face was bright, his eyes clear, and his voice enthusiastic as he offered me an option I'd never heard about.

"An epidural blood patch," he called it. "I'll just take some blood from your arm, here," he said, straightening my right arm and looking hungrily at the vein. The guy was earning a high *B* for salesmanship, but I had to hold off on his final grade until I'd actually had the procedure. "Then I'll take that same 10 cc of blood and inject it into the place in your spine where you had the anesthesia. The patch will stop the leak," he said, "and the headache should disappear."

"We can do it this afternoon," he said. He clearly loved his work.

I hesitated. I found the concept unnerving and even a little repulsive. I wondered if I should call Jeff to get his opinion, but the resident was waiting for an answer. In truth, I knew that if I talked to Jeff, his thinking would be logical and his response would be to the point: "You have a headache. You don't know how long it will linger. This could make it go away. Why not try it?"

The resident had barely left before an orderly arrived with a gurney, and I soon found myself rolling through what seemed to be the bowels of the hospital. As I lay on the stretcher en route to the anesthesia department, I managed to conjure up any number of reasons not to have the blood patch done. When the young doctor arrived with a tray of sterile equipment but no assistant or supervisor, he said, "We'll just roll you into this room and lock the wheels of the gurney. You don't even need to move to a table." He helped me with the awkward turn onto my side and then maneuvered my legs and upper body until I was in the position that he wanted.

I stuck out my arm as directed, and the doctor washed the skin with Betadine, wiped the Betadine away, and then wrapped a tourniquet up above my elbow. He patted around for a vein. I am not usually squeamish about needles, but the one he was about to use was a large bore needle like the ones the Red Cross uses to take blood. He was good, though, and hit the vein on the first stick and held the needle steady as dark venous blood filled the 10 cc tube. Since he had been competent with my arm, I felt a little more confident about him moving to my spine although I had a nagging feeling he was a little too excited about doing this. Plus, there was no attending physician hovering over him. See one, do one, teach one, I thought. I felt as if I might, in fact, be the "do one."

With the syringe full of the maroon liquid, he moved around to my back. I could no longer watch and had to supervise by feel. He swabbed my back with more Betadine and warned me about what was coming next. He moved his gloved fingers along my spine. Press, roll. Press, roll. I felt him thinking, counting. There, he decided. I felt the burn of the needle between my vertebrae. I thought about being paralyzed from the waist down, wondered how often it happened. I wondered again which number patient I was. Was I his first to do alone? Or number ten? I wiggled my toes every few seconds to reassure myself that the wires in my nervous system were still connected.

The whole process, from my conversation with Gayle to my return from the anesthesia department, took less than two hours. When I arrived back in my room, Gayle helped ease me back into my bed. She asked, "How's the headache?" I hadn't expected an instant result, but I moved my head experimentally, turning it from side to side.

"I think it's better," I said, hardly believing the pain could disappear so quickly and more impressed with how intuitive and quick this nurse had been. The ache was just barely there in the back of my head, a distant echo of its former magnitude. I turned on my side, thanking Gayle, appreciating the skill of a good nurse, thinking I was ready for a nap. Within moments I was asleep.

That evening, Jeff arrived with an armload of the items he thought I needed to keep me going for the week. I filled him in on the events of the preceding eight hours. Though it had been a day when a fluffy mountain of tissues had overflowed my wastebasket, at least the pain in my head was only a memory. He helped me out of bed and eased me into my robe and slippers. With Jeff's arm around me for support, we walked slowly down the hall to visit our baby in the neonatal intensive care unit.

WEEK ONE

Though Sarah's heart was still beating one day, then two days, then three days after her birth, there was not much going right for her. She had been born a perfectly formed and normally developed twenty-five-week fetus, but once her umbilical cord was detached from my placenta, she moved into a world she was not equipped to meet. Unplugged from her life-source, the baby-who-should-still-be-a-fetus had to breathe through lungs that were fifteen weeks away from being ready to work on their own. Her stomach and intestines were not mature enough to process milk, not even breast milk. Veins as fine as thread illustrated the map of her circulatory system under skin that was almost transparent. The bones of her skull were so soft that, if she were left in one position for too long, her head began to flatten to the contour of the surface it rested on. She had moved from a floating existence in the perennial dark of a mother ocean to a bright white place where the force of gravity held her down on the flat of a table. It took the latest-breaking knowledge and technology to substitute for an environment that had been completely natural in my body.

By Wednesday, day three, as the effects of pain medications were wearing off, so was my initial shock at Sarah's birth. I shuffled into the unit at around eleven that evening. I wanted to see Sarah before I went to bed for the night. I moved under my own power. My temperature was back to normal. I had no IV, a regular diet, oral antibiotics, only Tylenol for pain, and no further fainting episodes. As I worked my way down the aisle, I saw nurses standing in pairs beside isolettes, each evening nurse with clipboard in hand as she reported to the night nurse. Visitors were not usually allowed in the unit at change of shift, but the nurses didn't enforce that rule while I was still a patient. When I arrived at Sarah's spot, I could see the night nurse had already started her work. Clipboard in hand, she was sizing up the scene like a pilot at an airplane's instrument panel, assuring herself that red and green lights were flashing and alarms were set where she wanted them.

I stood by the table, looking at the baby, not touching her. I had not yet touched her. It still seemed that touching would be dangerous, and there was hardly a spot that wasn't covered with gauze or tape or Saran wrap. There was nothing cuddly about the baby in front of me. She looked raw and unfinished as if everything must hurt.

The night nurse looked at me for a moment. "Have you thought about having her baptized?" she asked gently.

41

I looked directly back at the nurse, but I couldn't speak right away. I wondered, is the baby worse? I couldn't tell. How could the nurse tell? Sarah looked exactly the same to me. Is she going to die tonight? I wondered. But I couldn't ask the questions.

"No. We haven't had her baptized," I finally said.

I hadn't thought about baptizing the baby. That was something people did when the baby came from home the hospital, wasn't it? They threw a party and dressed the baby in a long white dress and a frilly cap. Christenings were as important as weddings in my extended family. With seven siblings of childbearing age on my father's side and my mother's four brothers and sisters, it seemed there was always a christening.

I first became aware of the significance of baptism when my sister Elaine was born. I was six years old. Mom and Dad said the new baby couldn't ride in a car until she was christened. "If anything happened to the baby before she is baptized," my mother explained to me, "her soul would not be allowed into heaven. Her soul would go to limbo forever."

Even then I couldn't understand why a little baby could have the shadow of sin on her soul.

I am the product of a Catholic education. I attended Saint Joseph School from kindergarten through grade three, St. Martha School from the third through the eighth grade, Our Lady of the Angels Academy through high school, and for nursing I went to Boston College, a Jesuit school. Nevertheless, I had not been to a Sunday mass in a number of years. I never made a conscious decision to stop attending church. I simply drifted away. When I started my first job as a nurse and moved to a suburb of New Haven, I attended a local mass a few times, but the priest was worn-out and uninspired. As one sermon followed another, I heard nothing that stimulated my mind, touched my heart, or stirred my soul. So, with rotating hospital shifts that included working all hours of the weekend, I fell out of the habit of weekly attendance. For his part, Jeff had no strong feelings about religion, though he did attend church services as a child. Once they'd finished their pancake breakfast, Jeff's mother dressed and spit-polished her five children for their weekly attendance at the services of the Presbyterian Church in Wilmington, Delaware. Jeff's history of church attendance was less committed than mine. "As a teenager I went to whichever church needed a shortstop for its team," he told me, "or where there was a young woman who needed an escort to Sunday services."

In spite of our weak affiliations with organized religion, we wanted some kind of ceremony for Willie when he was born. We didn't need a name to attach to a specific faith, but we were looking for a spiritual welcome for our son. When we left Wenatchee with a car full of suitcases and two dogs, our first stop had been at Glacier National Park where our friends George and Kate lived. George was a lay minister who had performed the marriage ceremony for Jeff and me at Artist's Point in Yellowstone two years earlier. He seemed like the perfect person to baptize our baby boy.

We squeezed four adults and Willie in his seat into the car and drove to George and Kate's favorite stream in Glacier Park. They knew a spot just a short walk from the famous Going to the Sun Highway, a road that wended its way through and around the ragged mountain peaks formed by the movement of ancient glaciers. We pulled off to the side of the road and walked single file into the woods until we heard only the rippling of water over rocks and mid-afternoon bird talk. George knelt down and scooped some water from the stream. He played a cleansing trickle over Willie's head, and our son was christened William Going-to-the-Sun Blomstedt.

Of course Sarah should be baptized. She was in desperate need of a welcome into the world and whatever protection the light of God could offer her. So, the day after the nurse asked me about baptism, I called the hospital chaplain.

"Hello," I said. "I am on the third floor. I delivered a premature baby on Sunday and wondered if she can be christened by a Catholic priest."

I had assumed there would be a hospital priest, but the chaplain, who was not Catholic, gave me the phone number of a local priest. I called the number and repeated my story to the priest. Instead of offering a few words of comfort or understanding, however, the voice on the phone asked, "Why don't you call your own priest?"

A hot tingle erupted on my skin. I hadn't expected to be quizzed on the state of my own faith. I thought a priest would be pleased to have the opportunity to save a soul. I realized, too late, that because I had lived in Salt Lake City for two years, I'd confused the Catholic attitude towards baptism with that of the Mormons. The Mormons seek as many souls as they can for salvation, believing that unclaimed souls wander the universe until they are brought into the fold. They even convert the souls of those who are deceased. I had forgotten that the Catholic

Church required that the parents of a baby be active churchgoers and participating members of a parish in order for their child to be baptized.

"Ummm. I live up near Greenfield."

"Doesn't your priest come to the hospital to see people?"

"Well, I haven't lived in Massachusetts very long, and I don't know the priest in our town yet."

"What church do you go to?"

By then I was trembling. All of the feelings I'd had as a fifth grader in a pleated green-and-gray plaid uniform welled up, causing a wobble in my voice I could not control.

"Well, I don't go to a church there yet."

"Well, then. If you don't belong to a church, there is no point in my baptizing your baby. You have to join a church and have your own priest baptize the baby."

I didn't know what to say. I continued to hold the receiver to my ear but heard only the hum of the severed connection.

Alas, it was another day of crying. I cried in fear for my baby. I cried in anger at that priest and his sour soul. I cried at my disappointment in the Catholic Church. I cried for my sorry self. I cried because I missed Willie. I cried for Jeff, who was carrying the burden of his patients and Willie and me and the new baby. And then I cried some more, because I had no reason to stop.

The next day I woke up early and walked to the NICU before breakfast arrived. The day shift was about to take over. A nurse I hadn't met before was busy clamping, measuring, moving equipment and pushing buttons, but she paused from what she was doing and turned to greet me.

"The night nurse baptized the baby last night," she said without much preamble. "She looked at the baby's chart, and it said that you are Catholic. She hoped you wouldn't mind."

I felt my organs turn to mush. "No, that's fine," I managed to say. I was actually relieved and wished I'd thought to ask. In emergencies, any Catholic can perform baptism. "I'm glad she did. But was there a problem last night?"

The nurse shrugged. Summing up the scene with her look, she glanced at the baby, and I knew there was good reason for my insides to feel sick. The baby, like a tiny, featherless bird, lay stretched out on the warmer. She was attached to IVs, pumps, heart monitor, and breathing machine. I hadn't even held my child yet. I'd hardly touched her. The proper question was not, "Was there a problem last night?" What I should have asked was, "Is anything going right?"

All newborns lose weight in the first few days after birth, usually a few ounces. Sarah had no spare ounces to lose, but each day her weight dropped. The nurses reported Sarah's condition to us in neutral voices, but I could read unspoken meaning and unexpressed concern. Sarah's weight remained at 709 grams for the first three days, but that was because her kidneys were not functioning well. She was not urinating out as much as she was receiving intravenously, so the "stable" weight included water she retained. Lying under bright lights helped to bring down her bilirubin but also accelerated the evaporation of moisture from her skin. The doctors calculated how much fluid to give intravenously to make up for the losses. When her kidneys did finally kick in, the truth became apparent. She was losing weight. Day three: 680 grams. Day four: 595 grams. On day six she dropped even further to 539 grams, which translated to a number that was inconceivable: one pound, three ounces. She had started at one pound, nine ounces and lost six ounces in one week. That was one quarter of her body weight. She went down to nineteen ounces, just over a pound.

"How low can she go?" I asked David, Sarah's nurse. The complete question was, "How low can she go and still survive?" How small could the number shrink to and still, in the end, give us a whole and healthy baby who would crawl on the living room rug, play with blocks in her playpen, and step on a big yellow school bus that would take her to kindergarten? That was what I wanted to know. David shrugged, too uncomfortable to give me an answer. Her weight was about as low as they had seen in any baby who had survived. No one would say how much weight she could lose, still survive, and be whole. No one knew.

Sarah stayed at 539 grams for two days. She lived with lights, noise, the support of an endotracheal tube in her throat, IVs in her arm, leg, and umbilicus for fluids and medications, heel-sticks for blood, and even medicated enemas that drew out potassium that was rising to a dangerous level in her blood.

Finally, by the end of the first week, her kidneys began to function more efficiently, and she started to make urine that contained a balance of water and wastes closer to normal. So, the doctors informed us, her 539 grams—nineteen ounces—of body weight were finally real and not just water.

"We'll start giving her some calories intravenously within a few days," Dr. Rockwell said. Her digestive system was still not ready to take nourishment.

"When will she start to gain weight?" I asked him. "How long does it take a preemie to get back to her birth weight?"

"If all goes well," he said, "it usually takes about a month."

The doctor walked away, but his words hung in the air. I stood still.

This is something we should look forward to? I thought. A month to crawl back from one pound three ounces? In a month she will be back to just one pound and nine ounces? And where do we go from there? Will I ever see a seven-pound baby? When? Will she ever come home? I wanted to take the doctor by the shoulders and shake the answer out of him as if he could give it, as if my baby's condition were his fault.

The week moved slowly with Sarah dropping weight each day, hanging on one hour at a time. I sat on a maternal seesaw. At one end I needed to be with the baby. At the other end I missed Willie. Jeff took care of his patients and the home front, called me during the day, and visited each evening. His parents, whom we called Muz and Puz, came from Pennsylvania for a few days, and Muz kept Jeff going with a good breakfast each morning and the kind of suppers only a mother can provide. Each evening they came to the hospital to see me and their granddaughter.

I'd had other visitors. Sarah from family planning lumbered in one afternoon. She seemed hugely pregnant, her baby due in two weeks. It was probably hard for her to visit since the contrast in the outcomes of our pregnancies couldn't be more obvious, but I loved her for coming with her armful of flowers and a basket muffins. I received flowers from across the country, chocolates that melted in the US mail, and long-distance phone calls I didn't always want to answer.

By Friday I had been moved to a two-bed room with a young woman who told me she was in the hospital with hyperemesis, a condition of intense nausea and vomiting during pregnancy. She had been vomiting since the second month, she said, and I surmised she was in the hospital because the vomiting hadn't stopped. I swallowed hard, wondering if I would have to listen to her throwing up in the bathroom we shared. As a nurse that was my job, but as a patient, this was not the right roommate for me. With misguided good intentions the girl's family brought hot fudge sundaes for the two of us on Friday evening. What are they thinking? I wondered. Dreading the moment when my roommate's ice cream would reappear, I sat on my bed, twisting a spoon in the melting mess. It was time for me to leave the hospital.

Jeff had to make rounds at the hospital in Greenfield on Saturday morning, so when I was allowed to go home, it was my father who came to collect me. He set about gathering a cart full of flowers and the hospital supplies I had accumulated. When I prepared to take a shower, I realized all I had to dress in were the maternity clothes I had worn to the hospital six days before. I hadn't thought to ask Jeff to bring anything else, and while the clothes were clean, they had been sitting in a dark pile at the bottom of a plastic garbage bag and were a distinctly unappealing wrinkled heap of lost hopes. When I slipped into the balloon top and elastic-waisted pants and then looked down, I remembered seeing myself in the mirror six days earlier, expectantly dumpy, frumpy for a cause.

I looked in the mirror again. My face was pale. Dark circles under my eyes and limp hair reflected the confused state of my postpartum hormones. I was a disheveled mess.

Dad and I went to see Sarah together before we left. I took on the role of the professional tour guide, explaining how her machinery and equipment worked, telling him about her condition as clinically as one of the staff would have. What are you doing, Susan? I asked myself as I blabbered on to my father, but I couldn't make myself stop. I had to fill in the silence while Dad stood with his hands by his side, looking into the isolette, shaking his head. He had been in a few times earlier in the week, his face a sad reflection of the baby's condition. He would have visited more often, but I told him Mom and Willie needed him more at the end of the day. The truth was, I couldn't bear to see his sad face.

Standing there for the last time on Saturday morning as the mother-patient who was still emotionally joined to the baby-patient, I felt as if I were abandoning my baby. We'd come in together, but we weren't leaving together. I knew once I left the hospital I would be even less her mother and more like a visitor coming to look at her as if she were an animal in the zoo. Eventually, I stopped filling the air with words. I stared at the baby for a quiet moment, trying to hang onto her. She lay completely still, blindfolded and tethered to her equipment. Dad was very quiet.

Finally, I turned away. I'd talked to the resident about my medications and received my discharge orders from a nurse. Dad carried all of the paraphernalia down to the car. It was time for us to go, but I wanted to stay. I wanted to go. What I really wanted was to get to Enfield, hug Willie, watch him take the colored letters from the refrigerator and give them to Grandma, give him his lunch, put him in his crib for a rest, and then come back to the hospital so I could sit and watch over the baby for the rest of the afternoon. But that wasn't going to happen.

Dad and I didn't say much as we drove out of Springfield. The day was gray, but the cloud cover made the air less frigid than it had been on the previous Sunday. I looked out the window to my right at the Connecticut River where chunks of ice floated in a white-on-gray mosaic. The sky was gray. The river was gray. The snow on the side of the road was gray. I felt numb and empty.

I did not go back to the hospital that afternoon. I didn't have a car, I couldn't drive myself, and I didn't want to inconvenience my parents by asking them to drive me back to Springfield. I was not allowed to lift Willie per discharge instructions and needed help with him for at least a week while my abdomen mended, so it made sense for Willie and me to stay with Mom and Dad as long as they would have us. Jeff came later in the day with his parents. Mom made a lovely dinner, but the reunion was subdued.

Willie and I spent the following week with my parents, and either Dad or Jeff would take me to the hospital for a visit in the evening. Being unable to drive and seeing the baby for such a limited amount of time left me feeling severed from her. I was further muddled as I tried to figure out how I would arrange my life once I returned home. My heart was pulled by the force of the tiny life in the intensive care unit and the need to sit beside the baby's isolette, to talk to the nurses, and to see with my own eyes how she was doing in real time. I didn't want to get reports over the telephone. I wanted to be her twenty-four-hour private duty nurse.

But there was Willie. Which baby knows whether Mom is there for breakfast, lunch, supper, and all of the snacks in between? I asked myself. Which baby needs to see Mom first thing in the morning and for his goodnight kiss? Which baby needs a trusted routine? The answer was the same for each question—Willie. Jeff could pinch-hit in any of those places some of the time, but he couldn't do all of them all of the time and be able to work as well.

Visiting Sarah was something I needed, but my presence didn't help her. She lay in a technical cradle with a Plexiglas barrier between us. She was cared for by nurses who did what had to be done to keep her alive. She didn't know when I was there, and she didn't know when I wasn't.

But there was a little boy, warm, soft, and sticky-handed, who would be around no matter what happened to the baby, and he needed his parents. I also needed to be with Jeff. We would still need to hang together as a couple no matter what happened to the baby. As strong as my longing was to be with Sarah, I could not justify disrupting the routine at home by staying at the hospital day and night. After a week of wrangling with possible options, I came to the only conclusion that worked for me. I would spend some of each day as a visitor at the hospital, but my primary role was to be a partner for Jeff and a mother to Willie at home.

Two weeks after Sarah's birth, Jeff came to Enfield and gathered Willie, me, and the stuff we'd accumulated and drove us home. I walked into the kitchen in Gill, put down the few things I had been allowed to carry, and stood at the counter. All was neat and orderly after Jeff's two weeks of mostly bachelor living. The griddle from the Sunday pancakes was out of sight. The sameness should have been reassuring, but the quiet and dark seemed unnatural. Miss Weed demanded petting after so many days of being nothing but a dog. She was really an adult's dog but tolerated Willie and seemed to understand that his sprawling physical attentions would be short-lived. She allowed him to hug her around the neck and suffered through a few minutes of rolling on the floor. Then she retreated to a quiet corner where she could go back to being unnoticed.

An arrangement of flowers sat on the counter. I didn't open the card, did not even want to know who had sent the flowers. Their muted winter colors made me feel sad and empty. They made me think of funerals. My arms hung like weights by my side, and I didn't know quite what to do with them. I felt as if I'd gone shopping and left the grocery bags at the store or come back from a trip without my suitcase. The house and everything in it had stayed the same, but I was not the same. The woman who had flipped pancakes at that counter just two weeks before had disappeared.

The most pressing problem at home was making arrangements for Willie's day care so I could get to the hospital in the daytime. On Monday morning I started making phone calls. The woman who cared for Willie when I worked had no extra time to take him. After I pursued a few unsuccessful leads, my nurse colleague at family planning gave me the name of a woman who lived in Gill—Lynda. I dialed the number, and Lynda answered her telephone. I told her who had referred me and why, and Lynda murmured her sympathies. Then she said that as a matter of fact, she had Monday through Friday mornings available, but only until 11:30. We set up a time to meet.

"We are going to visit a woman named Lynda," I told Willie the following day as I zipped him into his red snowsuit. "She has kids playing at her house." I looked for some response, but none was forthcoming. "Can you say Lynda?"

I wondered how her name would come out. At eighteen months, Willie's word repertoire was limited. Most everything sounded like "dat doo." A cracker? "Dat doo." The big orange tractor in the garage? "Dat doo." Daddy? "Dat doo." The dog? Now, there was something different. "Weem!" he would answer, always with an exclamation point.

I asked him again. "Can you say Lynda?"

He was thoughtful for a moment. I thought he was going to pass on the question. But then he gave it a try.

"Yinna," he pronounced decisively even as he protested against the snowsuit's hood.

Good enough. He didn't have the L but his Y was working. We would head out and try it on for size.

When Willie and I walked into Lynda's kitchen, I felt as if we had stepped onto the movie set created for the Munchkins in *The Wizard of Oz*. The large open kitchen was laid out like a children's playhouse with everything from furniture to utensils arranged in a miniature tableau. The warmth that touched my face when I walked into the house was as inviting as the aroma of the banana bread baking in the oven. I knew right away I could easily spend all day with this woman. Her own children, Jon and Danielle, played with three others at a long, low kitchen table where they sat on shrunken chairs that allowed their feet to touch the floor. Lynda said she was about ready to bundle up her charges for some playtime in the snow. I couldn't imagine how. The morning was very cold, exactly like the day Sarah was born, the sun a dazzling force on white snow. I could barely get Willie dressed in boots, snow pants, mittens, and hats on winter days, but Lynda appeared to be unfazed by the prospect of dealing with six hats, six snowsuits, twelve boots, and twelve mittens.

Lynda had a space for Willie only in the morning because as a licensed daycare provider she could have only two kids under two years of age at a time. That meant I would leave him off at 8:30, drive an hour to Baystate, have an hour to spend in the NICU, and then drive an hour back. The time would be tight, but there was no doubt in my mind that the security I would feel as I left Willie with Lynda was worth the time restriction. At the end of the morning, Willie and I could have lunch, take a nap, and spend the rest of the afternoon together.

Keeping up a constant stream of four-, three-, and two-year-old conversation, the kids glued multicolored pasta elbows onto painted cardboard scenes. Lynda kept her eye on them, talked to me, and gently eased Willie towards the group. He found his comfort zone two steps back from the table where he stood observing the big boys with silent reverence. Paint, glue, scraps of paper, glitter. On the counter I saw piles of carrots and celery sticks ready for lunch. God bless her, I thought, and we signed up. Yinna it would be.

Sarah's condition continued to be critical, at first from minute to minute and then from day to day, but we never received a call saying, "She's in trouble. Come right away." There was no single crisis. When I visited the NICU, Sarah always seemed to be sleeping. The ambience of the unit was quiet and controlled, its orderly rows of isolettes lined up like cars in a parking lot. After the first week, once Sarah's condition stabilized and she was moved into her own isolette, she was yet another ongoing, but controlled, crisis. Because all of the babies were on ventilators, their breathing was assured, eliminating much of the potential for emergencies. Preemies in intensive care are different from adult patients in intensive care. Babies do not die from cardiac arrest. When they are in trouble, they are more likely to stop breathing. But NICU ventilators supported breathing and reduced the likelihood of respiratory arrest. Every bodily function was monitored. If a preemie was heading toward a crisis, the doctors and nurses knew almost before the situation showed in the baby's color or heart rate or muscle tone. Deteriorating blood values or a poor X-ray result gave them information ahead of time. There were few surprises although there were some problems even the most current treatments could do nothing to solve.

I never saw a baby die while I was there. I never heard one cry, either. It was eerie when I lifted my head one day and realized I had spent many hours in a room with eighteen babies, yet I had never heard one cry. Every one of them was on a respirator. Their vocal cords were separated by their ET tubes, preventing the formation of sound. One evening, I happened to see one of the babies in the middle of a crying episode. His tiny face was contorted with unhappiness. Or was it pain? I stood next to Sarah's box feeling helpless, unable to pick up the other baby or comfort him. If I'd been on a playground and someone else's child fell off the swing, I would have gone to him, brushed him off, wiped his tears, and helped him find his mother. In the NICU that wasn't an option. No parent stood nearby. The baby cried but made no sound. He was still too young to make tears, and that made his crying seem all the sadder.

They owe that baby some crying time when that ET tube comes out, I thought. Then I turned to my own silent baby.

When I visited Sarah on weekday mornings, I spent the first few minutes just standing in front of the isolette, sizing up her condition.

Then I quietly popped the latch of the porthole and slipped one hand inside. I hadn't held her yet—hadn't thought to ask since she was obviously so fragile and equipment-bound. Also, rather than being comforted by touch, Sarah often seemed disturbed when I touched her. I tried at first to stroke her, thinking that gentle, massage-like touch would be soothing in comparison to all the functional handling and painful treatments she experienced in a day. But instead of settling under my palm, she squirmed when I stroked her, probably because there was no cushion under her skin. I could see that physical contact did not feel good to her, but I needed to do more than just stand outside, looking at her as if she were on TV. Holding her seemed impossible, but I wanted to feel her. I wanted her to know I was there.

I learned to stop my hand from moving and instead let the weight of my palm and fingers mold themselves over her body. My hand covered her entire back, and once she got used to it being there, she would be calm. She would rest again, in sleep or whatever her state of consciousness might be, with an awareness that was not quite that of a fetus but not quite that of a fully developed newborn infant either. I could be with her for the hour then, and she seemed okay with the quiet weight of my hand. Sometimes a nurse pulled a chair up for me, and I could sit and talk to the nurse for the update of Sarah's condition while maintaining the connection between her little body and mine until my hand and arm grew numb. Sarah would lie quietly while my fingers tingled with the sensation of her spine and jutting ribs. I could feel the impossibly small movement of her mechanically controlled breathing.

If Jeff came with me, he would bend over to see how the baby looked and say a quiet "Hi, Little One" to her over the Plexiglas. He might reach through a porthole to rub her small head or pat her bottom and then move aside to let me in. He would check Sarah's chart for her weight and vital signs. Then he'd scan the room in search of a doctor or nurse who could give us an update on her condition.

One evening about two weeks after Sarah's birth, I sat with her while Jeff, restless, roamed the unit with hands clasped behind his back. There were no other parent visitors in the room, and I watched with mild curiosity as he peered into isolettes, looking at each baby and then the card stuck on each isolette. He bent over first one isolette and then another, each like a terrarium with its own variant of Homo sapiens growing within. I don't know if even he knew what he was looking for.

After ten or so minutes of this prowling, Jeff said, "Susan, come here!" His voice was excited. I sighed, not really wanting to "come here." But I lifted my hand from Sarah's body, gently closed the porthole door, and walked over to the corner where Jeff was standing.

"Look at this," he said, pointing to the Plexiglas.

I looked. In the isolette there was a baby on his tummy, his head turned to one side. I knew that the baby was a "he" because the card taped to his isolette was blue. He had what I recognized as the ubiquitous preemie look: elongated, flattened head, closed eyes, and face covered with tape. He looked like Sarah with more hair. From his mouth came an endotracheal tube wrapped with white tape that held it to his brown cheeks. I saw him tighten his lips and suck on the tube a few times as if it were a pacifier.

"So?" I didn't know what Jeff wanted me to see.

"Look!" He was pointing, emphatic. On the outside of each isolette the nurses stuck an identification card bearing the mother's name, the baby's name, and its birth weight. What Jeff wanted me to notice was that little José had been born in December at the same weight as Sarah, and he had finally, six weeks later, regained his birth weight. Jeff thought I should be excited by this fact. Another baby of Sarah's size had survived a month and looked, Jeff apparently thought, good.

The mere presence of little José, with his weight and significant dates recorded in ink on that ID card, was just what Jeff had needed to see. Always an optimist, he had been searching since Sarah's birth for a reason to hope his baby could survive. Now he beheld an undeniable fact in front of him in the form of a baby boy who had been born as small as Sarah and lived for six weeks. That baby's ability to endure became the rope Jeff grabbed and held onto. That little boy had made it, and as far as Jeff was concerned, so would his daughter.

Mystified by his excitement, I looked at him. I thought he was crazy, but I couldn't puncture his balloon with my gloomy thoughts. You think this is a good thing? I couldn't help but think. After six weeks in this place, six weeks of poking for veins, of having his heel pierced eight or ten times a day for blood, of transfusions, testing, and silent crying, this baby is only back to his miserable birth weight?

I kept looking at Jeff. My eyes wouldn't even blink. I felt disconnected from his enthusiasm and suddenly disconnected from him. I realized we were on different pages, in different rooms, on different planets, maybe, in the ways we were looking at our baby's situation. Two weeks after Sarah's birth, I couldn't stand the prospect of the weeks ahead, filled with the unknown. I felt as if I could handle anything, even her death, if I just knew what was going to happen. I had no words to say out loud, but the voices in my brain persisted.

A pound and a half after six weeks, I thought. God help you, little José. God help you, little Sarah. Then I finished the thought, and please, God, please help me.

LESSONS IN PHYSIOLOGY

Because she was born too soon, every system in Sarah's body struggled with its own efforts. Calculating and compensating for fluid loss seemed to be the number one challenge in the days after her birth. Fluids lost in the urine were measured by weighing her diapers. Fluids lost from her skin via evaporation had to be guessed at and calculated. Fluids lost from the lungs via the ventilator were replaced by the humidified air pushed in with each mechanical breath. The goal was to estimate accurately and then replace lost fluids without overloading her kidneys or her heart.

She was positioned on her back much of the time. Her arms were not curled up towards her face but lay stretched out by her side. Usually one arm was wrapped with gauze and attached to a tongue blade to keep the elbow from bending and protect the IV. Her legs were lax and quiet unless she was disturbed, and then she moved them only in response to discomfort. She was naked in order to expose as much skin as possible to the ultraviolet bilirubin lights she lay under for twenty-four hours each day. Even though I knew the temperature in the warmer was physiologically ideal, I felt cold when I saw her uncovered. Her unbabylike posture, her nakedness, her stillness, all challenged instincts that made me want to dress her and swaddle her and hold her close. We were obviously very far away from the day I might fulfill those simple, maternal urges.

Under the lights her skin turned an olive tone, but it became obvious as the first week ended that under the tan her skin had developed a yellow tinge. Even full-term babies become jaundiced after birth, but that process was magnified in Sarah. In the days after she was born, excess red blood cells that floated in her circulation started to break down. Bilirubin is a byproduct of those red blood cells. The liver is the organ in charge of detoxifying the bilirubin, but her liver became overwhelmed with the waste. Bilirubin circulated in her system and made her skin turn yellow. The solution in the NICU was to expose her skin to ultraviolet light, which was another way to break down the bilirubin.

The bilirubin level can rise quickly in a premature baby whose liver is not ready to handle the breakdown of red blood cells, and at high levels bilirubin is toxic to the brain. A few days after her light therapy was discontinued, Sarah's bilirubin rapidly spiked up to toxic levels again. When she turned a distinct yellow, the doctors ordered the therapy restarted with twice as many lights as she'd had previously.

Four fluorescent bulbs hung inside the isolette, where it was as bright as Fenway Park on a Saturday night. Under the heat of the lights, water evaporated from her skin at an increased rate, and the fluid-balancing act became even more complex. The doctors did not want to overload her circulation by giving her too much IV fluid, but neither did they want her to shrivel like a little raisin.

On the third day of her life, Sarah produced only three cc of urine. One measuring cup equals 240 cc of liquid. To visualize three cc, think of a medicine dropper and then squeeze out three drops. How did David, the nurse, even manage to measure such a minuscule amount of liquid? I knew he weighed every diaper before it was placed under her. Even a preemie diaper was so long beneath her it looked more like a mattress pad than a diaper. Then he weighed the diaper again when it was removed. But three cc?

To balance Sarah's accelerated fluid loss, she continued to receive carefully calibrated amounts of intravenous fluid. During my career in taking care of adults, the saying had been "One for a man, two for a horse" as we calculated medication doses. Compared to little kids I cared for in the pediatric ICU, the amount of fluid and medication measured out for Sarah was so small it seemed hardly worth giving. Because her kidneys were in shock and because she was so tiny, Sarah could tolerate only a little more than a half-cup of fluids in a twenty-four-hour period. I recalled hanging bags the size of a liter bottle of soda for my adult patients. Sarah's whole day of fluids could have come just from the liquid I would let drip into the wastebasket as I flushed air bubbles out of my patients' IV tubing.

While she was under the bilirubin lights, bulky white patches covered her eyes so I never could tell whether she was awake or asleep. Her skin was transparent. Each of her heels was a matrix of red commas where her skin had been jabbed and then squeezed for blood samples. But what made my gut twist more than anything was knowing Sarah was not getting any nourishment. Her weight decreased each day. I could count her ribs. All the body parts a newborn baby needed were developed but immature, and she had not even a molecule of body fat to fill in the spaces. To find a site for an IV, a nurse touched a flashlight to Sarah's tiny palm. She used the light that glowed red through skin as insubstantial as a plum's to illuminate the path of Sarah's veins. Her body was crying for energy, and there was some glucose in the IV fluids but not enough to grow on, not even enough to compensate for the calories she was using to survive the stress of a day. She continued to lose weight as she struggled with fluid balance, poorly functioning kidneys, and the immaturity of her stomach and intestines, which were not ready yet to digest anything. In hopes of being able to give something that might make a difference, I continued pumping each day. But she wasn't ready for breast milk yet. The stockpile of Baggies in my freezer grew, but my baby did not.

Most preemies suffer from respiratory distress syndrome, but Sarah's lungs had been spared failure or disease. The fatigue and achy thighs I had experienced in the two weeks before she was born had actually served a good purpose. The infection developing in my uterus set off alarms in my body that signaled Sarah's lungs to begin secreting surfactant, a slippery substance that coats the outer surface of the lungs and allows them to slide without friction against the tissues that surround them. Surfactant allows for the smooth, elastic, in-and-out of the spongy lungs, the expansion and contraction of breathing. Usually surfactant doesn't develop until the last few weeks in a normal pregnancy. Surfactant is often the variable that makes the difference in the survival of two babies born at similar weights. The one who produces surfactant has a significant advantage.

Sarah was attached to the respirator not because she needed high levels of oxygen pushed into her lungs but because the effort of breathing would have exhausted what little energy she had. Surprised at the low levels of oxygen she needed, the doctors told us her lungs were okay. I held on to that thought. With her kidneys floundering, gut unable to digest food, fluids evaporating, and bilirubin high, there was one hope. For now, at least, her lungs were good.

THE SHOEMAKER'S CHILDREN
HAVE HOLES IN THEIR SHOES

As expected, Sarah continued to lose weight. I wondered how Sarah's nurse David psychologically prepared himself to place her little body on the scale each morning. He recorded the decreasing number and watched her fade from little to nothing. The good news was, although her blood pressure remained very low, Sarah's kidneys seemed to be improving and her urine output was getting better. Although this made the neonatal team happy, it still challenged them in the delicate art of balancing her fluids. Her electrolytes and other lab values went up and down, but I had trouble interpreting the meaning of her weight each day. Increased weight could be a positive sign, showing she was on the rebound, but it could also be a sign of fluid retention or inefficient kidneys.

Over the first week of her life, I watched the name band identifying Sarah as "Baby LaScala" slip up and down her thigh until it worked its way down to her ankle and finally fell from her foot to lay abandoned next to her on the mattress. It was no bigger than a cigar band. She was unable to take any calories by mouth or by vein, gauze masks covered her eyes, and the fluorescent bili lights still blazed over her. She looked as if she had a severe sunburn. The fragile, thin skin of the twenty-five-week-old fetus was not prepared for exposure to light and air. Dried, cracked layers of skin peeled off the entire surface of her body in sheets as fine as a spider's web.

While the ventilator took breaths for Sarah on January 19, the second Sunday of her life, we held ours. Sarah was scheduled to have an ultrasound of her brain the next day. The purpose of the ultrasound was to check for hemorrhage, a common and potentially devastating complication in preemies. When I softly rubbed Sarah's head, the entire roundness of it felt surprisingly like the soft spot on a newborn's head. The individual bones of her skull were quite malleable. They weren't supposed to fuse at her stage of development because her brain still needed room to grow. The Caesarean section had reduced the trauma a vaginal delivery would have placed on the fragile neck and the soft bones of her skull, but hemorrhage was still a looming possibility.

On the night before she was due to have the second ultrasound, I lay awake, not sure I wanted to know if she'd had a hemorrhage. We had much to worry over but were still optimistic about her brain function because she wasn't showing any signs of bleeding in her brain. If she'd had a hemorrhage, we would expect to see paralysis or weakness in an arm or a leg, lack of movement on one side of the body, or changes in the pupils of her eyes. Staring at the ceiling, I still allowed myself the tiniest bit of hope that she would someday be a normal, healthy baby. The ultrasound result could wipe out my shred of positive thinking.

On Monday, January 20, Sarah weighed 539 grams—one pound and three ounces. It was the first day since her birth that Sarah's weight did not decrease. I held onto that good news on my ride back from the hospital that morning. By the time I arrived at home, however, I was mentally reviewing the risks of brain hemorrhage. I resumed worrying about the upcoming ultrasound and hovered near the telephone all afternoon.

Late that afternoon the phone finally rang. "Sarah had a normal ultrasound," Dr. Meyer said at the other end of the line. "The study showed no evidence of bleeding in the brain." I must have smiled. I certainly was relieved, but the overriding emotion was a confused kind of happiness. It was the kind of happiness that makes a parent want to sit down and cry after rescuing a child from the front end of a moving pick-up truck. I thanked the doctor for the good news, and we ended our happy conversation. After the initial relief, though, I wondered what Jeff and I would have done if the results had been different. How would we continue to support the aggressive medical care Sarah was getting if she'd had a brain hemorrhage?

When I worked in Yale's pediatric ICU, I found it heartbreaking to care for a child I knew would be brain damaged or handicapped, a child who was surviving only because of the extraordinary measures a large medical center could offer. One morning, a nine-year-old girl, Crystal, was brought into the pediatric ICU with severe head trauma. Her father was intoxicated when he drove her to school at eight o'clock that morning and took a corner too sharply. The car rammed into a guard rail and flipped over. Crystal wasn't wearing a seat belt. We did all we could for days, then weeks, to get her back. Neurosurgeons placed an intracranial catheter through a drill hole in her skull to measure brain pressure. We gave intravenous corticosteroids for brain swelling. A Swan line was threaded through the big vessels of her heart to monitor its function. Crystal received constant, measured, intensive care. Ironically, her situation became more frightening for me and the other nurses as her condition stabilized and became less critical because we waited each day for the thing that did not happen. We waited for the little girl to wake up.

Months later, after Crystal had moved from the ICU to the pediatric floor, I went to a mid-day picnic for the hospital's pediatric patients. The hospital lawn was populated with kids. I saw bald kids sitting with their moms, pale-faced kids pushing IV poles, laughing, healthy kids who ran in circles around their sick siblings. My friend from the pediatric ICU pointed to a young girl, alone in a wheelchair, who stared vacantly into the space in front of her. I didn't recognize Crystal—I had only seen her when she was unconscious with bandages wrapped around her head. Her arms rested without purpose in her lap. A nurse walked over to Crystal and began to spoon ice cream into the crooked mouth that opened automatically like a baby bird's. That little girl was the product of the pediatric ICU's lifesaving measures.

I wondered how the decision-making process worked in Baystate's NICU when a preemie experienced a brain hemorrhage. I knew the staff worked with professional commitment, but I wondered about their emotional dedication and the wisdom of giving time and resources to a baby everyone knew would be severely handicapped. After Sarah's normal ultrasound, I could push that worry to the side. With every normal ultrasound and each day Sarah survived, we moved farther away from having to respond to questions that had no easy answers.

The next day, Tuesday, Sarah's weight increased a bit to 567 grams, up by one-half ounce. I was buoyed by the news, but the following day the number had dropped again to 553 grams. The decrease was as minuscule as the weight gain had been, both probably meaningless, but I felt like a boxer who had finally stood up, a little wobbly after a punch, only to be knocked down again in the next round.

Anxiety plagued me. I read too much into every number, every lab value, every vital sign change, and my overly emotional reactions left me spinning without a center of gravity. I heard one report, and even if the result was good, I worked myself into a state of high anxiety while waiting for the next. I always believed that Sarah's situation was worse than the doctors were telling me. By trusting the negative, I was less vulnerable.

There was more news that Wednesday. I steeled myself, crossing my arms over my chest to take it. The bigger worry, the doctor said gravely on the day Sarah's weight dipped, was that she had developed a heart murmur. Sarah had developed a patent ductus arteriosus, a hole in her heart.

What else can go wrong? I wondered although I could recite a litany of bad things I knew.

When a fetus is developing in the uterus, the heart functions much as it will after birth. It beats in a regular rhythm to circulate blood through the fetus's body. The fetus has its own circulatory system independent of its mother's. While the fetus is developing in utero, the heart does beat. Because the fetus gets oxygen from its mother's circulation, the heart does not have to pump blood to the lungs to get oxygen. The developing fetus doesn't need to breathe air in order to be oxygenated, so blood circulates in a pathway that bypasses the lungs.

An amazing shift takes place at the moment of birth. When the newborn emerges from the birth canal, the opening between the heart's major vessels closes in response to the baby's instinctive urge to breathe air. The baby takes its initial breath. The lungs expand for the first time, and the heart makes a critical rearrangement of its circulatory pattern, moving blood to the baby's own lungs to gather oxygen. If that shift is not made and blood does not circulate past the lungs efficiently, the baby suffers from a lack of oxygen. In the short term, the skin takes on a bluish hue. Over time, the baby eats listlessly and grows poorly. If those symptoms are severe enough and if the circulation doesn't correct itself, the baby will need surgery.

To the doctors, the murmur detected in Sarah's heart was a disappointing but not surprising development. At twenty-five-weeks' gestation, the patent ductus arteriosus was understandable. For Jeff and me, it was a blow to hear such news after the week she had just struggled through.

The doctors said we had two options. "The first choice would be less invasive," Dr. Rockwell said. "A medication called Indocin. The protocol calls for three doses in three days."

I knew what Indocin was—an anti-inflammatory medication used to treat arthritis. How could it fix a hole in Sarah's heart? I had no idea, and it didn't much matter. It only mattered that it might do the job.

"We'll know after the three doses whether or not it works," the doctor continued. "If the treatment is successful, the patent ductus will close, and her murmur will go away. If not, the second option would be surgery."

They talked about taking Sarah to the operating room and fixing her heart. I glanced up at Jeff to see what he might be thinking. I wondered how they could seriously consider this option and listened to the doctors intently. I moved my eyes from one grave face to another. The procedure could not even be done at Baystate. Sarah would have to be transported by ambulance in a portable isolette to a children's hospital in Hartford or Boston. They were talking about a baby who had lost weight for a week, had bacteria infecting her blood from the moment of her birth, and needed one or two blood transfusions every day just to replace all of the blood taken for testing. They would have to move her into an ambulance with a portable ventilator, drive one or two hours to another hospital, take her to an operating room, put her under anesthesia, somehow manage to keep her alive with a blood pressure that could barely be measured, and then cut through her ribs to repair an opening between the chambers of a heart the size of a grape.

There was no doubt in my mind. If Sarah left Springfield, she would never come back.

I shook my head, not even looking to see if Jeff concurred. "Tell us more about the Indocin," I said.

The doctor sighed. "The Indocin is not without its own dangers," he began. "Indocin, as you probably know, affects coagulation. It prolongs bleeding time." The doctor continued. "Giving this medication will significantly increase the risk that the baby might suffer an intracranial bleed."

There it was again. All aspirins and anti-inflammatory drugs prolong the time it takes the blood to make a clot and increase the chance of hemorrhage. Bleeding in the brain remained everyone's greatest dread.

Though they put on brave game faces, the doctors didn't like the choices any more than we did. They decided to watch her for a week, to give her a chance to gain weight and see how her heart functioned while they worked through the possibilities. Though all agreed it was risky, surgery was an option they had to tell us about. I couldn't imagine my hand, or Jeff's, holding the pen that would sign permission for open-heart surgery. In my mind, it would have been the same as signing her death certificate.

Because her heart did not push blood efficiently through her body after the opening developed between the blood vessels, Sarah's fluid intake had to be restricted. When the doctor put a stethoscope to the baby's chest, he said he could hear crackles, indicating the presence of fluid sitting in the base of her lungs. That was bad enough, but more was to come. On day seventeen not only did the murmur persist, but a routine blood culture showed a new evil in Sarah's bloodstream.

Layered on top of her heap of troubles, cultures showed evidence of yeast, a fungus infection in her blood. To a baby of less than two pounds, the fungal infection was life-threatening. Other fungal infections, such as yeast in the vagina or thrush in a baby's mouth, are local, benign problems for someone who has a working immune system and is in good health. Candida in the blood of a premature baby like Sarah could overwhelm her systems and shut down her circulation, just as the bacteria in her body at birth had threatened to do. The only treatment for candida was amphotericin b, a medicine I remembered calculating into infant-sized doses in the pediatric ICU, a medication notable for its toxicity to the kidney.

Sarah began a course of amphotericin therapy that would have to be administered for six to ten weeks. The time frame seemed endless, and desperation hit me. Six weeks? I wanted to scream a primal, hair-pulling scream of maternal frustration and fear. Of course, it was obvious to any reasonable person who looked at Sarah that she would not be out of the hospital for at least six weeks, or ten weeks, or maybe twenty. Who knew? When the doctors talked about time—time for growth, weight gain, or for various treatments—I felt pushed to the edge of what I could tolerate. The times made me count days and weeks, and then I looked at the calendar. It would be March by the time she finished the course of anti-fungal medication.

Oh, my God, I thought, I can't last that long. The gnawing in my stomach will be a crater in six weeks. I yearned to see her as a bright-eyed, bouncing baby at some fuzzy time in the future, but no matter how I flipped the pages on my calendar, I could not find that date.

The inside of my head reverberated with a confusion of emotions: impatience with the doctors for moving so slowly to feed Sarah; a flash of anger at a nurse for slamming the portholes closed or not noticing an IV had infiltrated and was leaking into Sarah's skin instead of into a vein; craziness with Willie for acting like an almost-two-year-old; annoyance with Jeff, who managed to separate work and home in a way I couldn't understand; disappointment in myself for being unable to do anything but what I absolutely had to in order to get through a day.

I rarely looked at myself in a mirror, but I felt dull, lusterless, and washed out. I didn't wear any makeup. I couldn't pick up the phone to make an appointment for a haircut, and the layers of my December pre-holiday cut had melded into a limp straggle. I wore the same clothing every day, and I wondered if the NICU staff would suggest to Jeff that perhaps his wife ought to have a psychiatric evaluation before she completely lost her wits.

By the second week after Sarah's birth I didn't need my elastic-paneled maternity pants any more, but neither did my waistline quite fit into my pre-pregnancy clothes. After Willie was born, my belly had flattened in record time. I apparently burned up thousands of calories manufacturing milk for a lean and hungry baby, and by the time we drove out of Wenatchee, I was happily zipping myself into my old blue jeans. That didn't happen after Sarah's birth even though my belly was small when she was born. The artificial pumping kept my milk supply going but at nothing like the volume I produced for Willie. My belly wasn't shrinking. I was going out into the world every day, and I needed some new pants.

One Saturday morning in January, when Jeff was home with Willie and I had a little more time for my trip to Springfield than I did during the week, I decided I had to go shopping. I left the highway at Exit 15 in Holyoke and turned into the Ingleside Mall. The sky hung low, gray, and heavy, and the parking lot felt like a no man's land, vast and untrustworthy. I walked towards the entrance to G. Fox, a large department store. There had to be a pair of pants there for me.

I stepped into the retail universe. The air was different inside, not just warm but a packaged item all of itself. Light seemed to rush at me from every direction, as if on a stage set, bright light that bounced off a jumble of colors. My brain identified the atmosphere as disturbing. My eyes were not used to such light in the gray of that winter, and it almost hurt.

I stepped onto the uncarpeted yellow-brick-road that took me past each department but not into it, and I hoped that perhaps the slacks would find me. A woman wearing blue eye shadow, black eyeliner, bright red on her lips and lots of gold jewelry, sprayed a mist of perfume on the wrists of mid-morning customers. She turned to offer me a squirt, but I declined. Do people really believe that Calvin Klein perfume can make a difference in their lives? I wondered in my myopic state. Glass cases displayed an array of lipsticks lined up like soldiers in a pink and red army. Rack upon rack of lingerie filled the space on the left, nightgowns on the right. I was surrounded and enclosed by endless merchandise.

Suddenly it seemed there was far too much of everything, and none of it mattered. My chest tightened, and there was too much light and not enough air in the store. I needed to get out. I did an about-face without even touching an article of clothing, without having seen a pair of slacks on a rack, and pushed my way through the first doors I could get to. As quickly as I could without running, I found my way back to the safe familiarity of my car, unlocked the door, climbed in, and locked the door again. I sat for a while, letting my breathing return to a thoughtless rhythm, wondering if life had always made so little sense.

65

Some days later, still in need of at least one pair of pants I could zip and button, I tried again. At a small, local store I managed to find a pair of blue cotton pants in my new size. They fit, and I bought them and another pair in green. Each evening after that I took off one or the other pair of pants and hung it by a belt loop on a hook in my closet. I never bothered to fold the pants or put them in a drawer and washed them only when Willie spilled something on them or when I had worn them so long I was embarrassed by the tired wrinkles. I dressed in a long-sleeved plaid shirt that matched with both pairs of pants. In reality, no one at the hospital could actually see how I was dressed once I covered my street clothes with the white gown, but I imagined the staff must notice my unvarying look. By the time I dressed Willie each morning in pants and a matching shirt, I thought only about clean socks and underwear when I dressed myself. Having made those two choices, I reached for what I knew and came up with the same pants and plaid shirt, day after day.

Once the doctors learned that Sarah had candida teeming in her bloodstream, the option for surgery to repair her heart was off the table. The surgeons could not perform the operation on a baby with a blood infection, but neither could the neonatologists ignore the murmur because she was beginning to show some evidence of the inefficiency of her imperfect heart. Not only did Sarah have crackles in her lungs from fluid, but she was also beginning to experience episodes of bradycardia, times when her heart rate slowed and her oxygen levels dropped. She gave the doctors no choice. Something had to be done for her heart. On January 31, the nineteenth day of her life, Sarah received her first dose of Indocin.

While waiting, day by day, for the results of the Indocin treatment, the doctors searched for where the yeast infection had originated in Sarah's body. Fungi in the bloodstream spew from a nidus, a central spot of infection, often in the heart or the brain. After ultrasounding every organ, they found it.

"She has a fungal ball on her left kidney," Doctor Meyer told us. The irony of the finding was unavoidable. Sarah's father was a nephrologist, and his daughter was infected in the organ that he had spent his career researching, studying, and treating.

The shoemaker's children have holes in their shoes, I thought. The nephrologist's baby has an infection in her kidney. From an impossibly small spot on one kidney, a pinpoint of fungus spewed spores in all directions in the same way that spores spread from the underside of a mushroom. Microscopic organisms were floating in Sarah's blood, causing a fever and making her blood pressure plummet. The center of infection was a walled-off little spot, hard-bodied and protected from the outside against the anti-fungal medicines. I visualized it as one of the puffballs my cousins and I would discover in our grandparents' field when I was growing up, all hard and crackly on the outside and full of poof when we popped its crust. Under the best of conditions, it would take weeks of the amphotericin b to penetrate that outer coating. In Sarah's fragile state, I wondered how she would tolerate even the most carefully controlled administration of such a toxic medication.

I could locate Sarah easily when I walked into the unit. Amphotericin b deteriorates when exposed to light so the nurses had to cover the IV tubing and bag with aluminum foil in order to keep the medication in the dark. I just looked for her personal antenna, the silver tubing that wound its way down from the IV pump and into her arm. Because she had so few veins for IVs and needed other medications during the slow administration of the amphotericin, Sarah's nurses had to time the medicine so as not to interfere with her other drugs. Searching for an open IV line for the medication became a part of their daily routine.

Sarah looked the same from one day to the next, still like a featherless bird. She had not regained her birth weight, which seemed almost generous in comparison to her low point of one pound and three ounces. She needed two antibiotics plus the amphotericin, and the doctors increased the number of breaths from the ventilator because of the problems with her heart. With more breaths she experienced fewer episodes of bradycardia, but she also moved farther away from being independent of the ventilator.

Afraid to hope for good news, I walked into the unit the day after Sarah received the third Indocin treatment. Dr. Meyer was bent over the isolette, a stethoscope inserted through one of the portholes and pressed to Sarah's chest. I saw an unusual sight, a smile on the doctor's face.

"No murmur," she announced.

David, the nurse, nodded his head in agreement.

To reassure themselves that the silence held, they listened to her heart repeatedly while I stood there. The murmur had disappeared. Gone. They heard only the steady "lub-dub" of Sarah's heart without the extra swishing and swirling of blood in the heart's vessels. They let me listen.

"As her lungs clear, the episodes of bradycardia should decrease," the doctor said. Sarah's blood-clotting factors had remained stable while she was on the Indocin, and she showed no signs of bleeding. I called Jeff at work and gave him the news. For once we had a reason to smile through the telephone.

When I returned to Sarah's isolette, Doctor Meyer had moved on to deal with problems in other parts of the room. David was in the process of turning Sarah over in order to take pressure off her heels, buttocks, and elbows. He detached her ET tube from the ventilator for a few seconds while he gently repositioned her neck and made her comfortable on her tummy. Then he reattached the tube to the machine and closed the portholes on his side of the isolette. I opened one of the portholes on my side, lightly placing my hand over the bones of her spine. I tried to believe there was one part of this little person that I didn't have to worry about. Her eyes were closed, and she looked no different than she had on the previous days when the murmur whooshed in her chest. Mostly she appeared unchanged from one day to the next, no matter what the numbers said about bacteria, anemia, bradycardia, arrhythmia, or candidemia.

Looking down at her, naked and vulnerable, I knew with a feeling more familiar to me than the momentary happiness over her mended heart that Sarah was not even back to where she had started at birth. On that particular day she had leaped a single hurdle, but it was on a course where others stretched before her all the way to the horizon.

FLASH BULB MEMORY

My sense of the first weeks postpartum was of generalized numbness as if my entire person had been given an injection of Novocain. I couldn't feel my emotional limbs, couldn't identify my feelings, had to pat myself down every now and again to make sure all of my parts were in place. I don't watch much television, but public radio usually plays in my kitchen during the day, and news of the world sometimes filtered in through the numbness. I knew the New England Patriots were going to the Super Bowl not because I am a football fan but because the story was everywhere as if the voices of the sports reporters were floating on the Massachusetts air. While driving in the car, I heard a new song on a local radio station—"Sara"—by a band named Starship. Jeff heard it also, which surprised me since he was not known for being up-to-date on the top forty radio hits. He even went so far as to buy the forty-five record one day. He slapped it firmly on the kitchen counter as if a song bearing his daughter's name assured she would be a winner. We didn't pay much attention to the song's theme—it was a love song—or whether the words said anything relevant to our Sarah in particular, but I counted once and the name "Sara" was repeated twenty-three times in the song. We couldn't help but think it was meant for us to hear her name all those times, to keep her on the front burner of our thoughts as the song played on the radio each day.

On the national news front, I was aware that the space shuttle Challenger was due to launch from the Kennedy Space Center in Florida because I had been following the story of the teacher from New Hampshire who was chosen to be the first civilian to fly on a shuttle mission. Like everyone else, I was caught up in the drama of Christa McAuliffe's story, her training with the other astronauts in Houston, and her children and husband and the students in her classroom who were managing without her for a year so she could live the possibility of that American dream.

On the third Tuesday of Sarah's life, we bundled Willie into the car to take him to Grandma and Grandpa's so Jeff and I could visit the baby together. The temperature hovered in the single digits that day, and the station wagon was frigid from sitting in an unheated garage. Jeff eased the car slowly over the icy crust on our driveway, but instead of proceeding directly out onto Route 2, he pulled sharply left at the end of the driveway and directed the car towards the row of mailboxes lined up at

69

the side of the road. He knew without asking that I had probably not walked outside to get the newspaper or mail on that blustery day. After waiting for the electric window to screech its way down far enough for him to reach through, Jeff leaned over to open the door to the mailbox. Cold air rushed in through his window, adding to the creaky chill of what already felt like a freezer on wheels. He emptied the mailbox of its contents, handed the pile to me, then grabbed the paper from the next tube, and drew his head in. He pressed the button to roll the window up.

After the window was closed, Jeff placed both hands on the steering wheel but did not move the gearshift out of neutral. He turned to face me.

"Did you hear about the shuttle?"

"No." I thought about my day, the empty length of it. I don't know how I got through today, I thought. I didn't listen to the news. I didn't watch TV. The only conversation I had was with an eighteen-month-old child. "What about it?"

"It exploded after take-off," he said.

I looked at Jeff, my mind blank for a moment while the screen in my brain flickered and went black and then the power came back on again in a surge. He did not start driving while I sat with the news. The commentator's voice on *All Things Considered* droned quietly in the background on the radio, which had come on automatically when the car started, but I hadn't heard any of his words.

"The one with the teacher on it?" I could see fog from my breath on the air.

Jeff nodded without saying anything.

Then the Novocain started to wear off and pain crept into the layers beneath that day's numbness, like the feeling I'd had when my eight-year-old feet were frozen after hours of playing in the snow and just started to thaw in the warmth of my grandmother's kitchen. The hurt, when the warmth began to penetrate the skin, had been almost unbearable. The idea of the shuttle, the astronauts, the teacher, her students, and her family caused tears to well up so instantly they must have been sitting in a puddle just behind my eyelids all day, waiting for an excuse to be released. I could hardly get any words out. What was there to say? The lives of one teacher and five astronauts had been extinguished in the breath of time that separates one heartbeat from the next. "Oh, how awful" was all I could manage, trying not to see a vision of the explosion that insisted on playing in my head.

70

I turned up the volume on the radio as Jeff stepped on the accelerator and moved the car into the flow of traffic. One reporter after another dissected the emerging story. After some miles passed, their urgent voices drifted into the background again. My thoughts moved from the image of white smoke in a bright blue Florida sky to the black-blue of the ocean bottom where fragments of the airship now lay scattered to the dusky skin of my baby who was still a dream waiting to come true.

Jeff drove us south on the highway, and I could see the foothills in silhouette over my right shoulder. Within moments their shadows blended with the night sky. We rode without speaking. I felt so sorry— sorry for the astronauts, sorry for their families, sorry for the people who had looked trustingly up at a Tuesday morning sky. I searched through the glove compartment for tissues, napkins, something besides the back of my glove to use on my dripping nose. I turned to the back seat, knowing I could find something in the diaper bag. Willie was quiet, but his eyes were open, and he looked back at me. The car was warming up, so I turned all the way around and untied the string under his chin and slipped the red hood off his head.

"You're all bundled up there, little guy," I said. I thought of the astronauts as I lowered the zipper on Willie's jacket. I thought of the children who wouldn't see their mother again, ever. I found a tissue in the diaper bag. By the time I turned around in my seat and faced forward, I knew that the universal sorrow of that January 28 would cast a long shadow. It was one that swallowed up my own worries and made my little family's sadness seem very small.

ROLLER COASTER

On a February morning I woke to the vestiges of one of those vivid dreams that happen right before the alarm goes off. In the dream I had been forced onto an amusement park ride at gunpoint. I was locked into a seat with a chain around my waist and handcuffs on my wrists. Then the car was turned loose onto a track that never came into focus. For a while, Jeff sat in the car in front of me, but then the seat was empty and I had to crane my neck around to find him. He had no expression on his face. I grabbed onto him when I could reach him, or I clung to the bar in front of me, holding on with fingers gone white. Once when I reached for it, the bar wasn't where it was supposed to be, and there was nothing to hold onto for support.

The cars sped down the tracks and around the corners on two wheels on the verge of losing control. Jeff never made a sound. He did not scream when the track fell away and we dropped down, down until I thought there was no bottom. I opened my mouth to scream loud and long on the way down, but no sound came. It seemed if I could scream, I could make this thing stop. In the dream, I closed my eyes and held my breath as the car climbed up. In real life, I found myself in bed with my eyes open, staring at the ceiling, too afraid to move, paralyzed with the thought of starting another day on the family roller coaster.

Sarah's respiratory problems added to the complicated drama going on in her body. She began to experience more episodes of bradycardia and apnea. Bradycardia is a slowing of the heartbeat; apnea means "no breath." Those words became a new part of the report that the nurses gave when Jeff and I called or went to the unit. "She had only three bradys today," the nurse might say. Or, on a bad day, "She's having a lot of bradys today."

It seemed impossible that a baby who was on a respirator could stop breathing, but that was what would happen. The machine would breathe for her, but it was set to deliver a measured amount of pressure and a specific number of breaths to her lungs. The respiratory rate was set at fewer than the number of breaths Sarah actually needed each minute. She was not totally dependent on the machine to make her breathe—we knew that from her first cry—and she was supposed to take more breaths than the machine gave her. The hope was that she would eventually be capable of breathing on her own and would be weaned from the machine. She was getting ten or twelve puffs of air per minute from the machine. She took the other twenty or so she needed on her own power.

From one day to the next, the doctors tested her maturity and energy by adjusting the number of breaths the machine gave her. Sometimes, though, she did not do what she needed to do. Breathing doesn't happen just in the lungs. The brain regulates the urge to take a breath. Her nervous system was immature and did not consistently regulate her breathing. When, out of exhaustion or a chemical imbalance, she gave up the effort and did not take as many breaths as she needed, her oxygen levels would drop. Then her heart rate slowed down. Then it slowed down some more.

I was sitting in a chair beside Sarah's isolette one February morning, hoping her dark eyes would open for even a few minutes of my visit. As often happened, David said Sarah was tired by the time I arrived. She had been through her early morning routine: in and out of the isolette to be weighed; a visit from the respiratory therapist for a treatment to her lungs; medical rounds when the attending doctor, residents, and nurses gathered around her isolette and discussed her case. They examined her and wrote orders for the day. It was exhausting for Sarah, and she had dropped off to sleep. Though she didn't do much when she was awake—just lay there with her eyes open—at least I felt there was someone inside of the body when I was able to look into her eyes. I hoped maybe she could see me, too.

On that particular morning Sarah was resting on her tummy, head turned towards her left shoulder as obligated by her tubing and machinery. Mindful of each of the vertebrae that touched my palm, I had been sitting with my hand resting on her back for a while. After I'd had some quiet time with Sarah, David said it was time to change her position. I stood up, took my hand from Sarah's back, and stepped aside. David slipped his hands through the portholes and then eased them under her body. He supported her head and maintained its position with his right hand while he turned her body over with his left. Watching that procedure always made my stomach flip as it brought to mind the scene in *The Exorcist* when the girl's head rotates 360 degrees on her neck. I'd seen other nurses around the unit turn the babies in the same manner as David was turning Sarah, and the human neck does turn that way. It just always looked creepy to see Sarah's body turned over while her head stayed still, as opposed to seeing her lift her head up and turn it to the other side under her own power.

Sarah's eyes opened with unhappiness at the disruption of her sleep. As I moved to the other side of the isolette to be out of David's way, I became vaguely aware that the beep . . . beep . . . beep of the heart monitor had dropped off in its tempo. I hadn't realized how much attention I inadvertently paid to the sound. All at once, for no reason I could see, the baby wilted in David's hands. The sound of her heartbeat slowed even more, and as her heart rate slowed, her lids drifted down over her eyes, but they weren't sleepy eyes. They were eyes that were losing consciousness. Her arms and legs sagged as if David had accidentally pulled the plug on her body's energy source when he'd turned her. Within seconds, just one in and out of my own breath, Sarah's skin color changed. Even with so much of her face obscured by tape, I could see her lips had lost their shade of rose and her eyes seemed sunken under lids that were also blue. Her face had blanched to cold white. Suddenly the high-pitched alarm on the heart monitor rang out, but we didn't need the noise or flashing red lights to tell us there was trouble.

David quickly put Sarah down on the mattress and flicked the bottoms of her heels with his fingertips. The sharp discomfort should have caused her to take in a breath, but she lay limp and gray. Both the heart and ventilator alarms blasted in a piercing disharmony that made me want to clap my hands over my ears. Another nurse appeared.

"Ambu her, would you?" David said without looking up from his ministrations. Lauren slapped the alarms into silence. She knew Sarah because she had been assigned to Sarah on David's days off. Lauren disconnected Sarah's ET tube from the ventilator and attached the tube that came from Sarah's mouth to a connector on the ambu bag, a rubbery black bellows that allowed the nurse to puff air into the baby's lungs manually. Wordlessly, the two nurses worked over the baby. They showed no signs of panic, didn't holler for a doctor, and I wondered if their behavior was contained because I was there. Were they really as in control over the situation as they appeared to be? Puff . . . puff . . . puff . . . puff. Lauren's fingers worked in a barely perceptible motion as they squeezed the black ambu bag and caused the baby's rib cage to rise and fall as oxygenated air was forced into her lungs. Lauren kept her eyes fixed on the lengthened pattern of lines that indicated Sarah's heart rate on the monitor. Usually I could see a whole parade of squiggles that represented the Q-R-S waves of Sarah's heartbeat, but when the heart rate had dropped, only three or four complexes spread across the monitor screen.

"Come on, Sarah," I heard David say. I wished I had a job to do other than standing there, holding my own arms and watching the nurses as they worked through their maneuvers. How much time had gone by? A minute? Three minutes? I couldn't tell. Sarah continued to lie limp and unresponsive. Lauren rhythmically worked the ambu bag while David, moving Sarah's head and fiddling with the placement of the endotracheal tube, adjusted her position.

"Come on, Baby," he urged in a low voice. "Pick it up. You can do it."

Puff . . . puff . . . puff . . . went the ambu bag. And then something changed. The beep . . . beep . . . beep of the heart monitor started to increase in its rate.

Beep . . . beep . . . beep . . . beep . . . beep . . . beep. I couldn't take my eyes off the baby to look up at the monitor, but I knew the squiggles filled the screen again as the music of her beating heart sang in my ears. I hadn't recognized how much life Sarah had in her small body until I witnessed the stark contrast brought on by the bradycardia. Color was returning to her face. She didn't come back to the cherry-red nose of a kid who had just spent a winter afternoon sledding in the backyard, but with the return of oxygenated blood, her skin was infused with a hue that was at least compatible with life. When her heart rate increased, Sarah's fingers flexed and knees pulled up as if she had just awakened from a prolonged sleep.

Lauren reattached the ET tube to the ventilator and closed the doors on the isolette's portholes. David reset the alarms on the cardiac monitor and said, "Thanks, Lauren." Sarah was plugged in once again, the lights on the equipment were flashing, and all systems said go. The two nurses straightened up but did not look at one another or at me. They knew too much to allow themselves a smile over their small victory.

Then it was my turn to deteriorate. My backbone sagged, and my legs lost their strength. My heartbeat had to catch up to wherever it had left off at the beginning of the episode. I didn't know until it was over that my entire body had been shaking.

That was the first bradycardia episode I saw. Repeated incidents of apnea and bradycardia increased the downward speed on the February roller coaster rides. Sometimes Sarah would have four or five episodes in a twenty-four-hour period. The doctors changed the position of her ET tube and adjusted doses of theophylline, a medicine used to stimulate her breathing, but she had good and bad breathing days regardless of the maneuvers. Every time they changed the ET tube, she would have to have a chest X-ray to check the tube's position. That would make me anxious, thinking she would develop leukemia or cancer one day from all the X-rays. Then I'd catch myself. We'll be lucky if she lives long enough to worry about that, I'd think.

After the speedy downward ride, there was the slow climb up on the roller coaster. Sarah's minuscule weight gain, or the lack thereof, made me want to slip my fingers into my hair and pull. Sarah was over a month old when they finally started to feed her. Her weight was stuck at one pound and three ounces. The team of doctors didn't agree about what to do with feedings. From the day she was born, little brown smears of stool on Sarah's diaper consistently tested positive for blood. The blood was microscopic. There was no frank red color in the stool, but the tests remained positive. Blood in the stools can be an indication of necrotizing enterocolitis—NEC, they called it—which is a devastating intestinal disorder common in preemies. Just as her heart wasn't ready for life outside of the womb and her lungs weren't prepared to support her on their own, Sarah's intestines were not ready for the work of digestion. In NEC, blood supply to portions of the intestine is interrupted, and that tissue becomes necrotic—it dies. Once necrosis has occurred in the intestine, the only solution is to surgically remove the segment that has been destroyed. Keeping Sarah's intestinal tract empty by giving her intravenous nutrition for the first month of her life allowed the intestine to mature. The plan was for feedings to start very gradually when there was no sign of blood in her stools.

There was a second possible explanation for the blood in Sarah's stool. Her airway was chronically irritated from the ET tube, and blood from the irritation could be passing through the stomach and intestines and out into the stool. That seemed like a plausible explanation for the blood especially since her abdominal X-rays appeared normal and her intestines showed no sign of getting worse from one day to the next. Still, the doctors didn't want to take the risk of feeding her too early. The problem with continuing on the IV feedings was that the TPN—Total Parenteral Nutrition—could not provide enough calories for her to gain weight without also creating havoc with her kidneys and electrolyte balance. She was threatened by lack of nutrition. She stood between the proverbial rock and hard place.

When the doctors finally decided that they would try to feed her, I heard the words I had been waiting for since the La Leche nurse came to my room the day after Sarah's birth: "Can you bring in some breast milk tomorrow?"

"Can I?" I had been pumping and storing milk four times a day for five weeks. When the nurse asked me to bring the milk, the mother in me pictured baby Sarah sucking on a little bottle, but the nurse part of me knew that the baby really could not suck on the nipple of a bottle with the ET tube still in her mouth. Even so, a vision of her getting milk—my milk, painstakingly rendered— gave me hope.

The next day, when I delivered my cooler filled with little frozen packages of milk, the doctor said that feedings would start at one cc of half-strength breast milk every two hours.

"What?" I said, laughing a little, thinking he was teasing. One tablespoon of liquid equals fifteen cc; one cc is equal to about one drop from an eyedropper, and only half of that would be my milk. "One cc? You're kidding."

He wasn't. I tried to keep the disappointment from my face since the doctor thought he was delivering good news. But I was visualizing the little bit of milk I'd dribbled on the countertop when I filled Willie's plastic sippy cup at breakfast that morning. That puddle seemed about equal to what Sarah's calculated intake would be for the entire day. Even worse were the orders that the baby could not be given her next feeding if there was any fluid left in her stomach two hours after a feeding. Liquid left in the stomach meant incomplete digestion. Incomplete digestion could indicate problems in the intestinal tract. My own stomach churned. Of course there will be something in her stomach, I thought. Isn't there always acid in the stomach, some little bit of liquid? She can handle it. Give her a chance. But they were very conservative, very careful. The feeds were slow. The weight gain was minuscule. I was beside myself.

The rules of the feeding protocol were a torment. Her feedings were given by nasogastric tube, not by bottle yet, because she still had the breathing tube in her mouth. Once again, an activity as simple as sucking on a bottle would have used up too much of the energy she needed for growing. Instead of drinking from a bottle, Sarah had a tiny, pliable tube inserted through her nose and down the back of her throat into her stomach. The tube was also taped to her cheek, which was already covered with tape or the ugly gray adhesive from old tape that the nurses couldn't remove without abrading her skin. Her face was a mess, and as the days of February passed, she seemed to be sprouting more, instead of fewer, tubes.

My freezer at home was overflowing with frozen lumps of breast milk. The freezer had two shelves, and while the top level held peas and ice cube trays and a crystallized carton of long-forgotten ice cream, the entire bottom level was taken up with Baggies full of white liquid. I continued to pump whenever I could and almost always made the goal of four times a day. The pump was set up in the downstairs bathroom, and I usually sat on the floor while Willie wandered in and out or sat on the rug next to me and made drooly engine sounds to accompany the back-and-forth of his plastic construction vehicles. Unfortunately, that room was also the coldest in our drafty house, and I dreaded the process of peeling back layers of clothing to expose my chest to the cold air. The feel of the hard plastic cup against my breast and the sound of that motor represented everything mechanical about Sarah's life.

I had visualized bringing a few bags of milk to the NICU each day and pumping more to keep up with Sarah's needs. But that's not how it went. Sarah could take in very little volume, and her first oral feedings were a breast milk and water combination easy for her to digest. She needed less than an ounce of milk a day. The thawed breast milk would have to be discarded after two days. I brought in more milk, not because my previous delivery had been used up but to replace what had been thrown away.

When I thought of the nurses dumping each Baggie of two-day-old milk down the drain, I could hear my mother's words to my sisters and me when we were kids at the dinner table with cold peas and congealed gravy on our plates. "Think of those starving children in Biafra," she said, admonishing us to eat up. My ten-year-old imagination conjured up photographs I'd seen on UNICEF posters where solemn eyes stared at me. My adult vision was of silent African babies suckling from their mothers' shriveled breasts, and I wondered how I could put those hungry people together with my freezer bulging with bags of milk. I could take care of the children from an African village all by myself.

THE HIGHWAY

Forty-eight green mile-posts mark the length of Interstate 91 as it follows the Connecticut River Valley through Massachusetts, and every day the tires of my station wagon entered the highway between miles 42 and 43. I exited thirty-five miles later after passing mile marker 8. Though there were many places I could have visited on the way, I rarely made any side trips on my commute to the hospital. The time span from when I dropped Willie at Lynda's to when I would have to pick him up again was too short, and my interests had narrowed to what I could bring into focus through a pair of maternal binoculars. Often I didn't even turn the radio on, or if I did, I would search for a station, set the dial, and then never hear a song or an advertisement after that. One day I tried to listen to a book on tape to fill my brain with something other than worry. But concentration eluded me, and my mind left the story, the car, and the road.

I wished the trip could have fulfilled my need for a relaxing, reflective two hours each day, but I never achieved anything close to mental peace. On the way to the hospital I was rushing—rushing to get to the baby, to see her, to touch her, hoping I might find her bigger and better than the day before. On the way home I was rushing to Willie, to see him, sure he needed me. In those irrational moments, I was certain my little boy was too young to be left in day care each day. The speed limit was fifty-five miles per hour, but my right foot pushed the pedal towards the floor while my eyes furtively sought the hidden blue of state police vehicles in places I had seen them lurking on previous trips. I set the cruise control at sixty-two, but my foot pressed still harder as my impatience spurred me on to get there, wherever there was. One morning I passed a car with a bumper sticker on its fender. It said: "Beam me up, Scotty." That's what I need, I thought. Scotty's beam. The problem was I didn't know where I wanted to be.

Worse than the build-up of anxiety was the direction my thoughts traveled as I moved towards my destination. No matter which way the car was going, my thinking went downhill. When there was no real person within touching distance, I would think of Willie's smile and his new word of the week; Jeff's perspective and ability to find the positive; the physical bit of a baby, sleeping on her tummy. Then the ogres came. I imagined Willie scarred by a mother gone too much and too sad when she was around; Jeff gone to be with someone who was cheerful and fun;

and the baby blind, deaf, and brain-damaged. No one was with me in the car to dispute the thoughts that overwhelmed me, to walk me backward through the maze I would create.

Because I often stayed with Sarah for a few extra minutes, I had to make up time on the highway in order to get to Willie on time. I sped up Route 91 but then consciously slowed down to drive Main Road in Gill. I forced myself to leave the swirl of gloomy thoughts in the car as the tires crunched over Lynda's icy drive. One morning, running late, I rushed up the stairs to Lynda's house and then took a moment to peek through the window panes of the kitchen door. With a little plastic cup of milk and sections of a peanut-butter-and-jelly sandwich in front of him, Willie sat at the table in his green corduroy overalls. He quietly munched on a triangle while the other kids reached for carrots and ate their own sandwiches. On another day, working on a block-building project with Jon, his idol, he sat at the same table. Far from being upset, Willie was so engrossed in his play that he didn't even bother to look up when I opened the door and walked in. He was fine. He was happy. He had friends at this place.

Once I had company for the ride to Springfield. Lisa was part of a support group for parents of premature babies. She called me to introduce herself a few days after I'd come home, and she called me a few times each week. I knew she was trying to be supportive, but I found the calls more draining than helpful. I reverted to being a nurse as I explained Sarah's condition to Lisa, and that felt like a burden. Lisa was so curious. So interested. But the timing of the call was inevitably inconvenient or the thought of a fifteen-minute conversation exhausting. I knew I was being antisocial, but for whatever reasons, Lisa's phone calls did not make me feel better.

Lisa and her children came to visit Willie and me at home on a February morning. We all sat on the floor of my living room while the kids played. Once we caught up on Sarah, I had nothing else to say, so I asked questions about Lisa and her family. During the conversation, Lisa offered to keep me company on a future drive to the medical center, so we set up a time for the following week. I didn't know how to say, "No, I don't want you to come with me," and I thought there must be something wrong with me. I was feeling unfriendly and ungrateful, but the whole relationship seemed like work.

It will be good to ride with Lisa, I told myself. Instead of getting mired in black and blue thoughts on the ride, I will have the chance to get to know her better.

On the night before the planned trip, Lisa called and said, "I'll have to bring my kids, Susan. I hope you don't mind." I did mind. I cherished my adult time. I had only three hours without Willie each day.

"That will be fine," I answered, a fraud. "When should we rendezvous?"

We met at a parking lot in Greenfield on the way to the hospital for both of us. We decided to take my car. After getting the little girls out of their car seats, transferring the seats to my car, and resettling everybody, we were off. The conversation went in fits and starts as Lisa tried to manage the activity behind us.

Do I need this, I wondered once again, well-meaning as it is?

During a lull in the back seat action, I asked Lisa how premature her own baby had been. Her preemie, the older of the two, was three years old.

"Oh, she came three weeks early," Lisa answered very earnestly.

"She was three weeks premature?" I repeated, to be sure that I had heard correctly. "Did you have a difficult birth?"

"Oh, no, it went pretty well," Lisa said, and there was pride in her voice. "The birth was a little early, and my labor was difficult, so she was on a ventilator for twenty-four hours and then needed oxygen for a few days after that. They kept her in the hospital until they knew that she could tolerate her feedings."

"Oh," I said, mystified now about why Lisa was my contact from the support group. I repeated the numbers to myself: the baby was born three weeks early. Sarah had been born fourteen weeks early. To my mind, a support person was someone who is offering support out of a shared knowledge of a similar experience. From what she had described, the birth of Lisa's baby sounded nothing like Sarah's.

The baby must have been very small, I thought.

"How much did she weigh?" I asked, thinking that would be the answer to why Lisa was my support person.

"She was five pounds and three ounces."

"Oh," I said again. I heard myself speaking civilly but had to restrain myself from saying out loud, "You must be kidding."

Lisa turned to deal with fussing in the back seat. The kids covered for my silence. I couldn't stop my thoughts, ungrateful and unreasonable as the thoughts might be. What makes her think she can be a support to me? How can she say she understands? How dare she presume her baby's situation was anything like Sarah's? How could she possibly know how I feel?

I felt lonelier than I had on any other drive.

For Lisa, going back to Baystate was a reunion with the medical staff, and she had looked forward to the visit. When we arrived, Lisa wasn't allowed to see Sarah—no visitors were allowed in the NICU except for parents and grandparents—so one of the nurses who remembered Lisa and her child came to the parents' room to visit. Knowing Lisa's kids would get restless after a short time, I did not stay with Sarah for very long that day. My visit turned out to be even shorter than it usually was. On the way back to Greenfield, Lisa bubbled with enthusiasm for her visit. Feeling like a horrible human being, wishing for the solitude of my everyday ride, I moved us down the highway as quickly as I could.

After our hospital trip, I kept the phone calls with Lisa brief. I felt as if the relationship was all wrong. Lisa was as awed by Sarah's situation as everyone else was. That was no help to me. I thought the support group should have matched me up with someone who had delivered a baby like mine, someone who could understand the technology, the fear, and the black hole of time where I lived. On a bad day I should have been talking to a mother who could say, "That happened to my baby, too, and it was awful. I know how you feel," and really mean it. I was well aware there were very few parents of babies born as small as mine who could be part of such a group. Most babies who were Sarah's size did not survive. But a thirty-seven week baby hardly qualified as a premature birth, and I did not have the reserve of patience and understanding I needed to appreciate Lisa's efforts. As Susan the nurse, I could clearly see that, to Lisa, her baby's birth had been every bit as frightening and traumatic as Sarah's birth was to me. I knew Lisa was offering her time and a sympathetic ear out of the goodness of her heart, and I should have been more appreciative. But I wasn't wearing my nursing uniform. I was a mother, depressed, worried, antisocial, and unable to see beyond the bleakness of my own situation.

In contrast to the resentment I harbored towards my unsuspecting support person, the selective functioning of my brain did not cause me to feel anything negative towards my friends who called from Salt Lake City, Wenatchee, Grand Junction, and Burlington and who wanted to know all the details. I probably did not judge them as I did Lisa because they were not pretending to understand how I felt. They couldn't imagine it, they said. Tell us all about the baby, they said. You poor thing, you must be miserable, they said. I made sure they knew everything, any detail they asked for, how scary the days were for me, and how tenuous the hold on life was for Sarah. Sometimes I worried that I sounded like Eeyore when I talked to them, and they would eventually get tired of my voice. "She's so tiny. She's so scary. It's awful to see her."

Jeff handled the friends differently. When the phone rang and we were both in the room, neither of us would move towards it. It was like a game of chicken. Finally, one of us would give in and pick up the receiver. When Jeff was the one who took the call, he would share a little bit about Sarah and then steer the conversation in a different direction. He seemed to want to talk about anything but the baby, and the way he interpreted her condition to our friends always seemed more positive and more optimistic than what I saw in front of me when I stood by her isolette each day. He didn't even see her today, I would think with resentment as he spoke with authority about her condition. By the end of the conversation I would hear him laughing. He would have turned things around so that the long-distance caller was doing the talking as Jeff skillfully drew out the latest news. How can he laugh? I wondered when I heard him. I couldn't remember the last time I'd heard something that made me laugh. I wondered how our friends felt when they hung up the phone after talking to Jeff versus talking to me. When asked by their spouses, "So, how is Sarah?" I wondered how they replied.

As I drove the highway south and then north, I mulled over the disparity between Jeff and me. The differences were apparent in our conversations with friends, in our attitudes towards Sarah's present condition, in our outlooks about her future. Which of us was right? Who was being more realistic? I added those questions, and my inability to answer them, to the endless list of things to worry about.

In the end, I preferred being in the car with my own dark and dreary thoughts. I led myself down paths that caused me to blame the doctors for Sarah's slow weight gain, argue with Jeff's optimism, and grumble my way along the road as snow melted and red-tailed hawks returned to sit on tall branches of the trees that bordered the highway. Winter hinted it might retreat from New England, and silhouettes of maple trees showed outlines of early buds against the variable skies. The natural world may have been moving towards the green of spring, but when I drove the highway to and from Springfield each day, all I could see through my windshield were the same old shades of gray.

A BUNDLE OF BLANKETS

A nurse who worked with Jeff in the dialysis unit offered to take care of Willie on an evening of our choice so Jeff and I could have some time together. On the afternoon of our planned date, I turned on the news. When I heard the weatherman's predictions for a big snowstorm, I called Sue, the babysitter / nurse, and suggested that we take a rain check on her offer.

"I don't care about the snow," she said. "My husband will be playing with his band tonight, and I'll be home alone. I'd rather come to your house."

We left Sue and Willie with the makings of a macaroni-and-cheese dinner, a mountain of storybooks, and plans for a Cookie Monster bubble bath. With all of that to look forward to, Willie made no fuss when we said good-bye.

A few snowflakes floated in the air as Jeff turned the car out of the driveway and onto Route 2. There was no place for us to go on our date, of course, except to Springfield. We needed to eat, eventually. That was something we still did. But movies, concerts, and visiting friends were activities in our past life.

The road was wet with snow that melted as it touched the tire-warm pavement, but it wasn't slippery. Jeff and I were quiet. We didn't have much to say to each other about Sarah as the days of her hospitalization wore on. We dealt with the problem or question of the day but didn't spend a lot of time processing thoughts or feelings. We sat with the quiet rather than fill the space, probably because the words would have been all too familiar if we said them aloud. We were pretty quiet in general. Jeff never talks much medicine at home, and he talked even less about his workday after Sarah was born, probably because he knew none of it much mattered to me. I don't know where Jeff traveled in his mind as the car moved down the road, but my thoughts played like a symphony written in a minor key, a dirge winding round and round on the turntable until the arm lifted, moved, and then started the same record from the beginning.

Exit 26, Greenfield. It is taking her too long to gain any weight. She looked very puffy when I saw her this morning, her little hands and forearms swollen and filled with water beneath her thin skin. She is over a month old now, and I haven't held her. I can hardly touch her. She hasn't regained her birth weight as they said she should. That was the goal: she should regain her birth weight by a month after her birth, but she has not. Treating the fungus ball in her kidney has probably held her back. According to the ultrasounds it seems to be shrinking, but amphotericin b is like poison if they give too much and won't work if she doesn't get enough. The difference between the two is minuscule. She has to be on it for ten weeks, which means there is no hope she will be out of the hospital any time before April. I can't imagine ten weeks of this medicine dripping into those fragile veins. It is so caustic that the IV doesn't last in one place for more than a day, and then they have to go poking for another vein.

Exit 25, Conway. She has no places left for IVs. What are they going to do about that? Yesterday I saw a nurse, the one they call when they need the IV expert, bent over Sarah's isolette. Her face was all concentration as she looked for a new vein on the baby's hands, arms, and then her scalp. She searched first with her eyes, then allowed the pads of her fingers to play over the baby's skin as if it were a fine instrument. I pictured the whorls of this nurse's fingerprints all over Sarah's body and wondered how many fingerprints have left invisible marks on Sarah's skin.

Exit 24, Deerfield. No vein on the scalp. The nurse's fingers moved on. The feet? No, nothing there either. Her arms, maybe, or her hands. The woman's patience was apparently endless. She strained to see the promise of a blue line before she would consider trying to insert a needle. That nurse stayed bent over the baby for an hour before she actually picked up the butterfly needle to attempt the venous stick. An hour. I loved her for that.

Exit 23, Hatfield. I broke into a sweat well before the hour was up. I can't stand to be there when Sarah has to have a new IV inserted. Sometimes I have to leave. That needle hurts, and Sarah feels it, no question about that. When the needle pierces her skin, her face crinkles, and she tries to draw her hand or foot away. She lies there, captive, without a break in her day, without a break in what has been her life so far, suffering touch that is, more often than not, painful. Her feet are smaller than my thumb, and her little heels look like ground meat, each of them macerated with razor blade cuts where the nurses stab and then squeeze out drops of blood. It happens again in two hours. And then two hours later. I have a paper cut on my index finger that has been bothering me all day. It opens every time I bend my finger. What must her heels feel like? She feels pain, and she cries. Her silent cry hurts me more than her voice would.

Exit 21, Northampton. What does her voice sound like? How can I know her without hearing her?

Exits 17-15, Holyoke. The tube down her throat; the IV that has just blown in its vein and is leaking into the skin around the needle; the bright lights; alarms ringing around the room. She jumps at the BAM! SLAM! of the two portholes every time someone reaches into the isolette to turn or move or adjust her arm or leg or tubing or to get another sample of her blood. Her life is torture. Is this worth doing? Is this right?

Exits 13-11, Springfield. Then we have Willie to worry about. The tantrum he threw in the grocery store yesterday. That was new. Are we paying enough attention to him? Are we paying enough attention to each other?

The album was long-playing, double-sided, spinning around with the same thoughts from one minute, one hour, one day to the next. I assumed Jeff had the same worries, and we wouldn't feel any better when we talked about them because neither of us had any answers for the other. There was no comfort in talk. We couldn't even make small talk. Everything seemed trivial.

So we were quiet on the way to the hospital on that February evening. By the time we reached Springfield, snow filled the air and covered what had been frozen mountains of gray along the edges of the road with a fresh coat of white that sparkled in the beam of our head-lights. Our boots left prints in the snow as we walked into the building.

We did our time at the sinks, five minutes when the only sound was of running water accompanied by the rhythmic scrubbing of soapy brushes over knuckles and fingernails. Like programmed robots, we scrubbed for the same five minutes. Then we dried our hands for the same twenty seconds and slipped our arms into clean gowns to cover our clothes.

Stepping through the doors into the intensive care unit continued to feel to me as if I were entering a sacred place, like a cathedral or a concert hall where a symphony was in progress. The beep . . . beep . . . beep of the heart monitors in the intensive care unit played in different tempos and with slightly different pitches across the room. Over time I learned what the alarms meant: heart rate too low, IV pump empty, ventilator pressure too high. The alarm that always played a trick with my mind was the one that sounded when a baby was detached from its ventilator. The high-pitched squeal was exactly like the timer signaling that a batch of French fries at McDonald's needs to be lifted from its greasy bath.

Jeff and I wove through the isolettes to the place where Sarah lay. The first thing I noticed was that her diaper was off. The skin on her bottom was raw and abraded.

Though I had learned in college that the cause of bedsores was poor nursing care, I couldn't blame anyone for Sarah's sore bottom. If patients are turned regularly and kept clean, the skin should not break down. But Sarah had absolutely no padding on her body, and she couldn't move herself when she was uncomfortable. When she was placed in a certain position, she was stuck there until the nurse moved her, limb by limb, into another position. She had very little strength or energy, and she couldn't change position when her elbow was rubbing on the sheet or if her buttocks were irritated. So in the previous week she had developed areas of erosion on her skin.

When we walked in on that February evening, Sarah appeared to be sleeping, as usual, but I noticed something new in the isolette. She was lying on a sheepskin. That would relieve some of the pressure problems. The pile was so high that it looked as if she almost levitated above its surface.

Though Sarah lay on her tummy with her bottom showing, I could see she was dressed for the evening. One day, nearly a month after her birth, I suddenly couldn't tolerate her nakedness. It seemed dehumanizing for her to be so exposed. I asked my mother for help. With great enthusiasm, because there was finally something she could do, Mom went to the fabric store and bought swatches of yellow, pink, and blue flannel prints. She found a bargain, paying a few dollars for scraps leftover from some other seamstress's project.

Knowing they would have to work around the outfits, I talked to a few of the nurses to find out what design would work best for a gown. If the nurses didn't like them, the gowns would just stay in a drawer, so their input was important. Three of them stood together and warmed to the conversation as they listed the specifications of the perfect preemie gown.

"It needs to open in the back," said one, reaching her arms up behind her neck as if fastening a gown of her own, "and it would be convenient if it tied with a ribbon or snapped at the neck," said the other.

"What about the IV tubing?" I asked, remembering what a mess it was with my adult patients on the medical floor as I tried to thread bags of IV fluid through armholes. "Whoops! Wrong arm. Whoops! We did it backwards. Whoops! Let's try this again." Dressing an adult with an IV was a confusion of tubing, bag, and IV board. Sometimes I would fantasize about twisting the patient's entire arm off at the shoulder as I used to do with my Barbie doll, slipping the gown on the body, and then snapping the arm back into place.

"The shoulder seams should close with snaps," said the third nurse, expressing my exact thought.

My mother sewed four outfits out of the flannel prints, and each day the nurses dressed Sarah as if she were their little doll. Mom designed the pattern as the nurses had suggested with open shoulder seams that closed with snaps, so if Sarah had an IV in her arm, the nurses wouldn't create an entry for bacteria by detaching the IV tubing. They could just unsnap the shoulder seam and replace it around her arm and the tubing. Mom had also managed, with a pair of strong reading glasses, fingers that cramped, and needles almost as narrow as toothpicks, to knit three pairs of booties. One pair was a pale green, and the other two were bubble-gum pink. If my mother had been masterful with the gowns, the pairs of tiny booties were the pièce de resistance. The booties were custom fit to feet hardly more than an inch in length. Sometimes I would walk in during a busy part of the day to find Sarah naked except for the pair of pink booties tied with narrow pink ribbon that was woven through the stitches at the ankle. Dressing Sarah in those booties was a fine motor job, but the nurses were tickled with them.

I still struggled to find the baby in her. It was hard to see who she was with the ET tube in place. Somehow, I always felt better when I saw Sarah wearing her nightgowns. When she was totally outfitted in a flannel gown, with a stocking cap on her head and booties on her feet, I could see a hint of the baby we might just take home with us someday, and I had to find satisfaction in that.

On that snowy evening, a nurse I'd never met was assigned to Sarah. I assumed I had seen all of the staff in the unit by then. I found myself dependent on the nurses, even more than on the physicians, as my direct line to Sarah. The nurses were the ones who monitored the baby's moment-to-moment existence. The nurses knew everything that was knowable about our baby and had to report and record all of it. Realizing it took an entire shift to understand the complexity of such a baby, I would become impatient at best and afraid at worst with a nurse new to Sarah.

Anticipating problems before they happened required both familiarity and skill, and a good nurse could see problems early. Apparently Jackie worked only on weekends, and I had never been in the unit on her shift. She introduced herself with a direct look and a smile and moved easily around Sarah's equipment. I immediately felt comfortable in her presence.

David, Darlene, and Lauren were the nurses assigned to Sarah on the day shift, and Pete was usually the evening nurse during the week. I trusted them completely. They had been with Sarah from the beginning, and they knew her. I selfishly wanted them never to take days off, even when David told me stories about his own little kids whom he, of course, wanted to see.

But what about my baby? I thought as David talked about his Saturday plans. I knew it was unfair even as the thought popped into my head, she doesn't get the weekend off.

When Jackie introduced herself to us, I did not feel the usual anxiety about having an unfamiliar nurse. She was older than the other staff. They seemed very young at times, too young to know how nervous they should be about doing this job, I often thought, remembering who I had been as a new nurse. Jackie looked to be in her forties and worked part-time but had long experience in the NICU, she told us. Her smile warmed the space around us as she conversed with Jeff and me.

Without pausing in her movements in the maze of equipment surrounding Sarah's isolette, Jackie asked, "Were you planning to hold the baby tonight?"

"Hold her?" I said as if she had spoken to me in a foreign language.

Jackie's expression altered at my response, and she looked at me and then at Jeff. It was hard to read what the arched eyebrows meant. I felt as if I had made some kind of mistake but didn't know what it was.

"You mean you haven't held her yet?" The sentence almost sounded like an accusation.

Jeff and I looked at one another. "No, we haven't held her."

Jackie's eyes looked at us, at me, held on. "Would you like to?"

My ears rang for a few seconds. Holding the baby seemed impossible, the wires and tubing attached to such fragility.

Did I want to hold her?

I don't remember whether I responded to her question in words or just thought the answer in a jumble of feelings that swept through me like a flash flood.

Did I want to hold her?

"Can she really come out?" I asked with more composure than I felt. "Isn't it too dangerous for her?"

Apparently Jackie didn't think so. She moved into action. First she fastened a diaper around Sarah's bottom and tucked the spindly arms and legs into a receiving blanket. Sarah was already wearing her booties, and Jackie eased a little stocking cap onto Sarah's head to prevent her from losing heat in the cooler temperature of the room. The transfer preparations turned into a complicated production of rerouting IV lines, connecting and disconnecting tubes, and muting the alarms so they would not ring. The endotracheal tube had to stay in place, of course, but Jackie wrapped an extra strip of tape around the tube and then safety-pinned the tape to the receiving blanket so the weight of the tubing would not pull on Sarah's face.

Jeff motioned for me go first. Another nurse, recruited for the project, dragged a big wooden rocking chair from across the room, turned me around, and positioned me in it.

Any number of times I almost changed my mind about holding her, not because I was nervous for me but because it was obviously such a big deal to do this to Sarah. It was a big stress for her to come out of her controlled environment. In the end, though, I wanted it too much. Forty-eight days after her birth into what had thus far been an unfriendly world, a nurse handed my baby to me.

There was no perceivable weight to the bundle. The holding seemed almost silly as if there were only a bulky wad of blankets in my arms. Yet the energy force of a life—my daughter's life, so rough in its beginning—lay close to me, and I was finally certain of its power. Through the flannel and beneath the tubing, her not-quite-round head, not much larger than a tennis ball, was wrapped in a flesh-colored stocking tied at the top with a piece of pink flannel string as if to keep any of her energy from leaking out. I looked at the little bit of her I could see—her nose and her eyelids, which she kept tightly closed. She didn't seem to mind the change once we were quiet together, and we rocked. I closed my eyes and rocked my baby.

Awaiting his turn, Jeff sat on the sidelines with tears in his eyes. After a period of time that was impossible to measure, we switched positions. Sarah looked ridiculously small in the cradle of her father's arms, and he looked ridiculously happy to be holding her. He never moved his eyes from her little face.

The atmosphere in the car on the ride home could not have been more different than it had been two hours earlier. There were silences, but something besides worry was going on in the quiet. Between the moments of reflection, we talked.

"There was nothing to her. It was like holding a bundle of blankets."

"Wasn't it weird? She weighs so little, but it was as if the blankets were filled with energy."

"I know. You're right. I felt it, too."

As the car crawled slowly north in what had become a swirling February snowstorm, we sifted through the events of the evening. Only one lane of the highway was open, but Jeff and I, father and mother of little Sarah, had no fear of the slippery road. We drove along at thirty-five miles an hour, but we were in no hurry. It was as if time stopped for the moment and Sarah's medical complications fell away. Our spirits had been plugged in and charged up by something powerful, a life force that weighed less than two pounds.

SIX STICKS OF BUTTER

While I spent the days dividing my time between managing the home front and commuting to see Sarah, Jeff left early for hospital rounds and a schedule filled with patients suffering the gamut of illnesses from colds and sore throats to heart failure, diabetes, and kidneys gone bad. At Franklin Medical Center, he was surrounded by people who wanted to know about Sarah. Aware that her condition changed from one day to the next, friends and colleagues wanted current information.

On the evening after we held Sarah, Jeff stood at the kitchen counter and stared into space. He processes issues internally before they make their way into conversation, so I didn't ask him what he was thinking. I swabbed the remains of dinner off Willie's face and hands and set him down on the floor. Then Jeff seemed to make a decision. He walked out of the kitchen and came back a few minutes later with a collection of what looked like supplies for an art project and piled them on the counter. There were a pair of scissors, white glue, colored markers, a Polaroid photo of Sarah that had been taken at the NICU a few days earlier, and an old button he had excavated from the far reaches of a desk drawer. I turned the button over. It was blue and said, "It's a boy!"

He picked up a pencil and began to trace the button's shape onto the photo. That done, he cut the photo into a round and glued the circle of Sarah's intensive care face, all tape and plastic tubing and tightly closed eyes, onto the button. He took up the scissors and the sheet of yellow construction paper, then snipped with small, careful bites. He pushed the scraps aside and wrote with a black marker on the yellow paper. He took up the glue and stuck the little paper sign to the bottom of the button.

He turned the button around so that I could see the completed project. The words on the paper said: "Six Sticks of Butter."

I looked at the button and then at him.

"Okay, I give up," I said, not feeling clever enough to play a game. "What does it mean?"

"That's what she weighed today," he said, pinning the baby-faced button to his shirt pocket and patting it twice. It was the day Sarah finally regained her birth weight. For the second time in her life she weighed one pound and nine ounces.

"No one can really conceive of her size," he said. He was right. Who could visualize what a baby looked like at a pound and a half? I could hardly remember what Willie was like as a newborn. How could anyone understand Sarah's size? And it seemed important that they did understand, that they respect her size and the power, both the technology and Sarah's own will, that kept her alive.

Jeff wanted to put Sarah's size in perspective. He is very good at such things. I suppose his ability comes out of his medical training, or maybe it is the Boy Scout in him. On the rare occasion when he does not have a tape measure in his pocket, he uses his own body parts to measure things. It might be the round of a fingertip, the length of a finger, the distance from the tip of the longest finger to the elbow, the reach of his outstretched arms, or the span of his stride. He then takes his measured body part anywhere, be it to a patient's medical record or to the hardware store, and converts his anatomical ruler to centimeters or inches or feet.

With his own daughter, Jeff was trying to describe weight. When his co-workers passed him in the hospital corridor in the winter of 1986 and saw the words beneath the baby's photo on the button pinned to his shirt pocket, he was answering their question—"How much does she weigh today?"—and teasing them with a puzzle. The hospital staff read the label—Six Sticks of Butter—and then smiled a little uncertainly and continued to walk down the hallway. Later, as they stood in the lunch line or delivered a film to the X-ray department, they tried to fit the pieces of the puzzle together. The moment hit when the X-ray technician or the nurse or the cafeteria worker or the physical plant manager connected the baby face on the button and the negligible weight of a few sticks of butter. They probably couldn't visualize what Sarah looked like from the numbers that described her, but in their minds they could see the little bit of space six sticks of butter occupy in a refrigerator.

Then they got it.

As eager as I was to get to the hospital and the baby as I sped down the highway each day, a heaviness settled over me—over my chest, if I had to pick a part of my anatomy—when I finally found myself checking in at the hospital desk. The heaviness came from having no hope that anything about Sarah would have improved from when I had called earlier that morning and nothing the nurse told me had changed from what I had seen in the baby the day before. The heaviness came from knowing she may not have suffered any disaster but neither had she made any measurable leap forward.

When I went to visit her, I had to wait in a holding room on the hospital's ground level before being allowed to pass through security to the elevators. After I signed in, the guard who served as the gatekeeper for the intensive care units would call up to the NICU to see if the situation in the unit was under control and it was an appropriate time for visitors. When he shook his head in the negative and told me I would have to wait, I never knew if the delay was because something was wrong with someone else's baby or mine. The waiting and not knowing made me anxious. Chafing at the loss of precious visiting minutes in the small window of time I had while Willie was at Lynda's, I sometimes had to wait as long as a half hour before the guard would give me the okay and I could go upstairs.

That dreary waiting room and the ambience of the old part of the Springfield Hospital came from a time when hospitals did not actively compete with one another for patients. Decor was not a significant item in their operating budgets. The color brown dominated halls illuminated by yellow light that never seemed bright enough. The smell was of musty antiseptic and a thermostat set too high, like the wing where I had worked at Yale-New Haven Hospital, a building of the same vintage. Sometimes I confused the smells in the present with smells from ten years before, and they were equally vivid. Instead of walking with the heavy footsteps of a thirty-one-year-old mother, however, the much younger nurse had walked purposefully in her white uniform and soft-soled shoes up stairs and along other brown hallways.

Though it was six years since I'd lived in New Haven, the walk towards the elevator that led to my baby could be disorienting at times. If I closed my eyes while waiting for the bell to ding and the up arrow to light over the top of the elevator doors, I could forget when I opened my eyes again where I was going and what button I was supposed to push.

A routine day: number forty-five. The elevator doors opened to the fifth floor, and I stepped out. I could hardly remember the woman who had slumped to the floor in that same hallway in the confused days after Sarah's birth. Six weeks later, I was strong of body but operating with limited emotional power as I turned left and then right, then pushed the button that opened the door to the unit's foyer. I hung my coat on a hook in the closet next to other winter parkas. I felt sad for their owners.

An anteroom divided the rarefied environment of the NICU from the rest of the hospital. It worked rather like the mudroom in my house, except that in addition to leaving bulky jackets behind before entering the unit, visitors and staff needed to shed their germs as well. The coat closet was on the left, and a row of sinks lined the wall on the right. Sometimes there were other parents or a physician scrubbing as I rolled up my sleeves in preparation for the required hand wash. I could tell if the parents next to me were new when we scrubbed side by side. Those of us who had been there a while worked at the sink as nimbly as the NICU staff.

After the speed of my drive down the highway, the brisk walk from the parking lot to the hospital building, the impatient wait for a nod from the security guard, and then more time spent waiting for an elevator to transport me up to the fifth floor, the time standing at the sink was the transition from one world to another. I turned my back to the coat rack and faced five minutes of scrubbing. I had finally arrived at my destination, yet it seemed like the hands on the clock stopped moving as my own hands performed automatically under warm water flowing from the faucet.

I pushed the plunger and squeezed a gob of Hibiclens, a pink anti-bacterial liquid, into my right hand. In my memory, most hospital scenes appear dream-like, a little fuzzy around the edges. But when I stood at the NICU sink and smelled Hibiclens, the color pink, like a tuft of cotton candy, filled the place behind my eyes where past hospital scenes played. In the Yale pediatric ICU, we nurses had to scrub our hands at the start of a day or an evening or a night of work. We repeated the activity a score of times each shift. We all had dry, chapped hands.

Here I was again, in scrubbing meditation, with soap smells and hospital gown confusing the past and the present. I used a brush to scrub over and around my fingernails, and a satisfying mound of pink-tinged bubbles formed on the backs of my hands, on my palms, and around my wrists. I rinsed off invisible bacteria from hands that had looked perfectly clean when I walked in. Then I pulled a clean gown over clothes that had just come from my dryer at home.

Before Sarah's birth, I hadn't felt sorrowful when I walked into a hospital. The medical center had been my workplace. As a nurse, I had experienced individual moments of sadness, of course, but my prevailing state of mind had been an edgy excitement. In contrast, when I scrubbed my way in to see Sarah, I felt gloomy. For each small improvement Sarah made, some other complication would set her back, and I honestly could not tell how the balance sheet added up from one day to the next.

On that February day of confused reminiscence, I arrived early enough to be with David, Sarah's primary nurse, when he weighed her. Getting her weight was an involved but necessary part of Sarah's routine. Her weight told more about her condition than any other number.

In order for Sarah to be weighed accurately, she had to be completely undressed. The equipment that surrounded and sustained her complicated what would have otherwise been a simple procedure. David flipped buttons up and down to turn off alarms on her heart monitor and ventilator and then removed clips that connected sticky pads on her chest to the monitor. When she was free of wires, he placed his fingers where her ET tube connected to the ventilator hose and deftly detached one from the other. She had no trouble breathing on her own for the twenty seconds it took to weigh her. Working quickly to reduce stress to her as much as possible, David slipped what looked like Goliath's hands underneath Sarah's body and swept the little bit of a person out of the warmed isolette. He pivoted and turned toward the scale. David and Sarah made an incongruous tableau when he did this. They exaggerated each other's proportions. He placed her gently onto the scale covered with a pre-weighed washcloth to protect her from the cold metal. She turned her head to one side and scrunched her face up so that it looked like a dried apple, her entire body visibly unhappy about the cool air and the hard surface of the scale. With skinny arms extended all the way up and over her head, she stretched, showing off all of her thirteen inches. She had not achieved much new length since her birth. My friend Ginny, calling from Salt Lake City, said she could not imagine the size of such a baby. I told her to look at the telephone receiver she was holding in her hand. When Sarah lay on her belly with knees tucked up beneath her, she was no bigger than that part of the phone.

When the weighing was finished, David reversed the procedure. Looking like someone who had just found a newly-hatched bird, he held the creature away from his body, turned gingerly, and returned her to her nest. He reattached all of the equipment and reset the alarms. Sarah settled again in her home. The excursion to the scale was her biggest outing that day. Her weight was recorded on a new flow sheet that hung on a clipboard near her isolette.

February 25, 1986. Day 45: 2.0 pounds. Another day for Sarah, and a new number for Jeff to write on his button.

MAPLE SYRUP

On a cold evening in March, one of Jeff's college roommates called from Vermont. Phil and his wife, Anne, phoned often to check on Sarah's progress and on ours. Jeff talked first, giving Phil a fair summary of Sarah's week. Then it was Phil doing the talking, and I heard Jeff say, "Oh . . . really? Yeah . . . yeah." He listened again. "Uh huh. That sounds great! Hold on, let me check with Susan." He covered the mouthpiece of the phone with one hand and turned to me. "Do you want to boil sap with Phil and Anne this weekend?"

The sap was rising in the veins of Vermont's maple trees. A stretch of cold nights followed by warm, sunny days had the clear liquid overflowing the buckets hanging in the woods behind Phil's house. He and Anne were new to sugaring, and they could hardly keep up with the volume of running sap. They knew they would be stoking the wood fire and boiling sap all day on Saturday and probably on Sunday, too.

I thought about it. A day with Phil, Anne, and their son Gordie sounded so appealing, so normal, a family adventure the likes of which had been nonexistent for us since January. But going to Vermont meant neither of us would get to the NICU on that day. It meant we would not get to Springfield at all.

"We can't do that," I said. "What about the baby?"

Jeff looked at me with a neutral expression on his face while he continued to hold the phone. I thought I knew what he was thinking. The baby's condition was stable. Yes, she was barely over two pounds. Yes, she was still being treated for a kidney infection. Yes, she was still on the respirator and experiencing daily episodes of bradycardia. Nearly eight weeks had passed since Sarah's birth, but it seemed her condition changed in ways hardly measurable from one day to the next. Nothing would be different that Saturday, either.

I looked out the kitchen window and saw nothing but my own reflection. I could not meet Jeff's eyes because I knew I was being irrational. We both knew how much Jeff, Willie, and I needed a day to move out of the oppressive atmosphere surrounding our lives. Our house was stuffy and claustrophobic. We needed fresh Vermont air.

Jeff probably knew he had the greatest chance of persuading me to see both sides of the issue if he said very little. He gave me room to argue both sides in my own head while he stood patiently, holding the phone.

"Okay," I said. "I've never boiled sap before. That sounds fun." Then, feeling as if I had made the right choice for us as a family but had betrayed my daughter, I walked out of the room.

We agreed to leave at noon on Saturday. Jeff needed to make rounds on his hospital patients in the morning, so I stayed home with Willie and no one went to Springfield. At 11:30, I called the NICU for the second time that day and, no surprise, there was no change in Sarah. Her weight was two pounds and three ounces. She needed the ventilator for breaths, but she no longer needed extra oxygen mixed in and was breathing room air. Her skin was puffy with retained fluid, and she was getting a diuretic for that. She needed more calories than she could take in through the feeding tube in her stomach, but they couldn't give her more of the hyperalimentation—a white concoction of lipids that dripped into a large vein near her heart—because, while the IV feeding helped her gain weight, the lipid mixture also contributed to her puffiness. Maintaining her fluid and electrolyte balance was a continuous challenge, but nothing in her condition, not even her weight, had changed from the day before.

We left home at a little past noon, driving north in the direction opposite of where I wanted to be. The morning had started off bright and sunny. The temperature was pleasant for the time of year, but by the time we crossed the border into Vermont, the wind had kicked up, clouds had settled over the low mountains, and my mood had deteriorated to match the gray. A few raindrops spattered across the windshield. Jeff did not touch the control for the windshield wipers as if the rain didn't exist while he could still see through the window. Willie was settled into his car seat behind us, getting friendly with a peanut-butter-and-jelly sandwich. His favorite singer, Raffi, played on the car tape deck. By the time we got to Brattleboro, tears were welling up in my eyes faster than I could swallow them. They finally spilled over and ran down my face. Droplets poised on the wool of my sweater.

What is wrong with me? I wondered. Why am I never happy when I am in either place . . . with the family or with the baby? I felt a physical pulling as if Sarah and I were still attached by some imaginary umbilical cord, as if the long green tubing I'd seen hanging from the maple trees that lined the roads in Gill was connecting Sarah to me. Now the tubing was stretching, thinning, and pulling tighter from deep within my body, and it was about to snap. I wasn't sure it would stretch as far as Arlington, Vermont.

Looking out the passenger window as if I were fascinated by the scenery, I could not see through the blur. I felt Jeff's look.

"Are you crying?" he asked.

I sniffled in response, not turning my head to look at him. It would be some years before I read *Men are from Mars, Women are from Venus*, and I was unaware Jeff and I did not always interpret each other's words correctly. Not only that, I was expecting him to read my mind. On that afternoon in my as-yet-unenlightened state, I could not believe I had to answer his question. It was inconceivable to me that he didn't instinctively know we should not be going north, that I would be miserable if I did not see Sarah that day, that it was irresponsible for us to expect to do anything that might be fun while we had a baby who lay in the hospital struggling to hang onto a life we gave her and she never asked for.

I didn't answer him, so he tried another question.

"Do you want me to turn around?"

More sniffling. Then I really had to make a decision. I ran the film in my head. If I said yes, turn around, which everything in me longed to do, I visualized us getting home and me driving down to Springfield in a frenzy, rushing into the NICU. I'd find Sarah in the same time warp, lying in the isolette exactly as she'd been when I visited her on the previous evening. Not smiling up at me with recognition, happy to see her mommy. Just lying on her tummy, eyes closed, respirator huffing, monitor beeping her heart's rhythm. I would stay for an hour, maybe two, and then would turn around to make the return trip up Route 91. Phil and Anne would be disappointed but understanding.

I could have that day, or I could spend a brisk March day visiting with our friends. I knew I was being overwrought and unreasonable, but I felt guilty that I might enjoy a day while Sarah suffered through hers in the hospital.

While I processed these thoughts, we passed the first Brattleboro exit with one more to go before we turned onto the next leg of our trip. I faced forward and looked through the window in front of me and silently admitted this day was important for us. We had drifted so far from center, from the days of singing duets to Jeff's ukulele as we drove hundreds of miles, from the puns and wordplay that started when Jeff scribbled in code on a napkin on our first date, from the quiet of shared intimacy so different from the wordlessness of our separate worry. Jeff and I probably needed this day even more than I needed to be with Sarah, and I had to face what I could not change. Her essential needs were still technical, and there was nothing I could do for her. I had to make another choice, as well. If we decided to get off at Exit 2 and head west on Route 30 toward Manchester, I would need an attitude adjustment as we used to call it on Yellowstone hikes when the trail got too long or the mountain too steep. I could not continue on this adventure as a morose and miserable spoiler.

I opened the glove compartment and rooted around, found a napkin, and blew my nose. I dried my face and then turned around to look at Willie. The little guy had fallen asleep, and I saw his long fingers, spread wide on the car seat, sticky with grape jelly. I turned back and looked at Jeff.

"Let's keep going," I said as we approached Exit 2. He reached over to squeeze my hand and then signaled right, turning the car into the curve that took us off the highway.

Though we had been to Phil and Anne's house only once since our move back east, I had no trouble recognizing their property as we approached it on the country road. Smoke drifted up from the weathered gray shack that sat not far from the road, and steam swirled around Phil's head as he peered out to see who was driving into his yard. His cheeks were flushed, and his long, smiling face reminded me of the Tin Man in the *Wizard of Oz*. He looked as if the makeup technician had slapped some high color on his cheeks to prepare him for the scene. Phil was shadowed by his five-year-old assistant Gordie. Anne walked out from the kitchen to join us. We hadn't seen these friends since the summer before Sarah's birth, and warm hugs moved from adults to kids and back to the adults again. Charged up by his nap, Willie was ready for action, and standing around and listening to adults talk was not his idea of fun. He turned toward a path that led into the woods. Jeff leaned on the shack and immediately started quizzing Phil about the details of his sugar-making operation. Anne returned to the kitchen, and I followed the boys into the woods. Gordie peeked into each bucket, which happened to be at just the right height for him. Until I moved to Gill, I had never lived far enough north in New England to see the clear drops of maple sap dripping from the tap, had never before heard the steady plink . . . plink . . . plink . . . of liquid hitting the bottom of an empty tin bucket. I crouched down and explained to Willie how these drops that look like water turned into the syrup that we poured on his Sunday morning pancakes. He looked at me as if I were telling him a fairy tale and then picked up a stick and poked at the pine needles where a chipmunk had just disappeared.

When the boys and I returned to the sugar shack, the guys were laughing at some shared story, and so the afternoon continued. The clean air seemed to expand my lungs and carry new energy to the rest of my body. I even laughed that day. It happened after hours of stoking the fire with wood, after the clear sap had finally boiled down to a rich, brown liquid. Darkness and hunger drew us from the sugar shack into the house, where Anne had prepared a Mexican feast. The food seemed especially delicious after a day in the late winter air. We ate Spanish rice and bean burritos topped with shredded lettuce, salsa, cucumbers, and sour cream.

My first plateful of food disappeared quickly, and I thought I would help myself to just a little more. Instead of interrupting Phil in the midst of the story he was telling, I reached over my plate and around my drinking glass to get the bowl of refried beans. With a serving spoon full of beans on its return trip to my plate, I lost my focus and the gloppy mess of beans slipped off the spoon and plopped noisily into my glass of ice water where it settled at the bottom. A few shards of brown swirled around and around in the water. No one said anything for what seemed like a long time.

Then Phil broke the silence. With a completely straight face he said, "Very appetizing, Susan."

The grownups guffawed. I laughed, probably too long and too hard, and laughed some more until the tears ran. I wiped my face with my napkin and blew my nose. Eventually the silliness stopped, and Phil excused himself from the table. He returned with a clear glass of water for me.

Jeff and I were quiet on the way home. The toddler-timing of this trip had been perfect both ways. Willie had been busy running around in the woods or adding kindling to the fire all afternoon. With a full belly, he dropped off to sleep almost immediately for the two-hour ride home in the humming warmth of the car.

Usually we took turns driving on such trips, but I was once again on the passenger side on the way home. I closed my eyes and reclined my seatback. The visit had been the right thing to do, of course. I couldn't get over the sense that the day was incomplete without Sarah, but the feeling I had was not the raw desperation that had overwhelmed me earlier. I was warm in the car and filled with fine food, funny stories, and a good kind of tired from the afternoon outdoors. I let the dark cover me like a blanket and thought about the day and the vision of steam rising from the bubbling syrup into the March air.

When we pulled into the driveway, the car's digital clock read exactly ten o'clock. Jeff looked over at me as the car idled in front of the garage.

"If you want, we can go to Springfield now."

I shook my head.

While Jeff carried the sweaty, limp little boy up to his crib, I walked into the kitchen and picked up the telephone.

Day Number 70 was about to be just another completed page on the medical records for Sarah.

"Nope. No change today," said the evening nurse. "She's been pretty quiet." Her weight was unchanged from the morning. I wondered if there was any way Sarah could sense that I had not been with her on that day. I'd read studies reporting that preemies know, as evidenced by increased heart rate and brain wave activity, when their mothers are present. No matter what the studies showed, though, in my heart I was sure of what I knew. My baby lay in a transparent box where anonymous hands moved in, out, and around her all day, doing what needed to be done to keep her alive. My presence in the hospital on that day would not have made her well or happy. My absence had not made a bit of difference.

I walked up the stairs and tiptoed in to give Willie a goodnight kiss. I breathed in his scent of sweat, wood smoke, and some kind of berry juice and wondered if Sarah would ever be here with us and sleep in her own crib after a day of play with friends. Still, my guilt about enjoying the day had diminished, and I didn't get overly morose. I stood watching the in-and-out of Willie's breathing and felt a lasting warmth inside as if I'd carried home some of the embers that glowed in the sugar shack's dying fire.

BOXING GLOVES

I suppose if I had made a sincere effort to compare Sarah's condition in March with the way she looked in the weeks after her birth, I might have been forced to admit her situation was improving. But because she improved so slowly and because I was constantly steeled against the next catastrophe that might develop, I was unable to look at her minuscule advances and see them as overall progress. Somehow I couldn't accept the idea that, since Sarah was supposed to be born in April, it was only natural she would be discharged from the hospital sometime in April. Why did I expect her to be ready to come home any sooner? Under any circumstance, she needed approximately forty weeks of growth in a controlled environment, and since she couldn't use my uterus for the last fifteen weeks, she would have to do it in an isolette.

The isolettes in the NICU impersonated the human uterus in technological form, and the intensive care unit was a microcosm that operated on its own timetable. The NICU ran on uterine time, a designation that was different from eastern, central, or Pacific time. The nurses and doctors were comfortable with this time frame. They were accustomed to the pace of uterine time and did not expect to see much change in their charges from one day to the next just as I wouldn't have noticed much change in my belly from one winter day to another had I stayed pregnant for the normal 280 days. Because the nurses worked on uterine time, they could see and be satisfied with changes in Sarah that I could not. I worried constantly about the slow progress in each of her systems. Her heart had repaired itself, but her kidneys were infected with fungus. Her lungs were moving air, but would her brain ever tell her to breathe on her own? She didn't need high oxygen doses, but would her eyes be normal? She required long courses of antibiotics, and gentamicin is known to cause deafness in children. For one of Sarah's infections, gentamicin was the only antibiotic that was effective. Could she hear normally? Was there some way to test that in a tiny infant?

I wanted my family together. I wanted Sarah home. And greedy mother that I might be, I wanted my baby, when she was ready to take her first steps into the world, to do it with every system at maximum power. I wanted her healthy in every way.

Sesame Street was the only TV show Willie watched, and it played at seven in the morning, during the noon hour, and from four to five o'clock in the afternoon. I would usually make a call to the NICU in the late afternoon when Willie was settled in front of Grover and Cookie Monster, and I knew the evening nurses had organized their work for the upcoming shift.

On a March afternoon, I cradled the phone on my shoulder as I started to take silverware out of the dishwasher and set the spoons, knives, and forks into their individual slots in the kitchen drawer. I noticed with surprise that sunlight still played across the frozen expanse of Barton Cove at nearly 4:30, a promise that we might see the end of that winter.

Sometimes the wait for a nurse to come to the phone was long. Sometimes the person who answered the phone put me on hold and neglected to tell Sarah's nurse I was on the line. Maybe the nurse heard but was distracted and forgot a call was waiting for her, and I would have to hang up and call back. I felt like a nuisance when I had to say, again, "Hi, this is Susan LaScala, Sarah's mom. I just called, but no one came to the phone." The ward clerk was always apologetic, of course. On that March afternoon, I managed to empty the entire dishwasher and set the table while I waited on hold.

When I was about to hang up and redial, I finally heard the voice of the nurse for the evening shift.

"Susan? Hi. It's Pete." She sounded a little breathless. "Sorry it took me so long to get here." My annoyance always melted away as soon as I heard a voice. I was glad it was Pete's. She knew Sarah's routine cold.

Pete said, "Sarah extubated herself this afternoon." Maybe it wasn't breathlessness. Maybe she sounded a little triumphant.

"She what?" I knew that to extubate meant to pull out the breathing tube, but that made no sense. I had seen Sarah earlier in the day, looking as she always did. I was so accustomed to getting the routine answer when I made the routine afternoon call that I was stunned to hear Pete actually had something new and surprising to report.

"Sometime between the last time David looked at her and when I did, she managed to sneak the endotracheal tube out." I pictured the scene even as Pete told the story. The baby lay in the isolette, apparently sleeping, while the unsuspecting David made his final notes on the clipboard. Surreptitiously, Sarah inched her right hand nearer and nearer the tube. Shifting her eyes side to side under half-closed lids, she curled tiny fingers around the white plastic, tightened her grip, yanked the thing out of her mouth, and tossed it to the side in disgust. Then she lifted her head, purposefully turned her face in the other direction in a way she'd never been allowed to do since her birth, and went back to sleep.

"She extubated herself?" I was repeating myself. I felt like cheering, though Sarah's pulling out her tube was risky. She hadn't spent more than five minutes off the ventilator in her short life. The safest way to get her to breathe on her own would be to wean her from the machine, not to stop it cold turkey. The plan was to give a decreasing number of breaths from the machine each day so that she could adapt by increasing the breaths that she triggered on her own. That process hadn't been started yet, so there was a danger that she could exhaust herself and stop breathing after she pulled the tube. The fact that she was showing her strength seemed like a good sign to me and, I think, to Pete, as well.

Finally I thought to ask, "How is she now?"

"Well, they reintubated her pretty quickly," Pete said, bursting my bubble of hope. "But she did real well breathing on her own for about twenty minutes while the ET tube was out."

The doctors told us Sarah would eventually be capable of breathing independently, but how could they really know? The opportunities for her to breathe on her own were very rare. They reinserted the tube because Sarah was still too small and too depleted to continue breathing independently. She needed to gain some weight before she could be freed from her tether. But at that moment I felt the same pride that I heard in Pete's voice. There was a person in that impossibly small body, and she might even be a little bit feisty.

The nurses seemed to have special affection for Sarah, but I didn't know what it was about her that made the nurses so attentive. I had trouble seeing the distinctions between one unformed NICU baby and another. If someone asked me if all the kids I had cared for in the pediatric ICU were the same, I suppose I would have been appalled at the insensitivity of the question. But the differences in the pediatric ICU patients were easy to see because we took care of kids who ranged from newborn to sixteen years. The premature babies, in contrast, seemed generic. Every one of them was tiny, nearly bald, and skinny, with prune faces hidden under white tape. They lived in identical containers and were so weighed down with equipment they could hardly move. They made no sounds. They did not smile, and they rarely opened their eyes. They didn't even have the option of being fussy. Sarah certainly was not cuddly in the way we expect babies to be, and neither were any of her roommates. They were a scrawny bunch, all bony protrusions and thin skin, and there was nothing even remotely cute, in the Gerber baby sense, about any of them.

Though the nurses shifted their patients' positions as often as they could, eventually all the babies' heads were flattened on the sides. They lay for so long with their heads positioned on one side or the other due to the restrictions of the ET tubes that the gradual change in skull shape was unavoidable. All the NICU babies should still have been floating bottoms up in a warm, amniotic bath, where the soft bones of their heads would expand in slow, gradual growth without pressure from any side. Instead, they were victims of gravity, the would-be roundness of their occipital bones weighed down months ahead of schedule. In addition to Sarah's flattened skull, her face obscured by white tape, and her bird-like arms and legs, she had a raised, cherry red spot on her forehead called a hemangioma. It measured about one-half inch in diameter and perched on the front of her head at the hairline, a little off-center. It wasn't of any particular concern, and the doctors said it would increase in size for a while and then shrink as she grew older. Yet despite what I thought of as undeveloped imperfection, there was something about Sarah, the nurses insisted, that was special. She was cute and she was a fighter, and they liked that.

When I walked into the unit scrubbed and gowned on the evening of the day Sarah attempted to lose her ET tube, she lay in her usual position with her eyes closed. Nurses from around the room drifted over to talk to me.

"Did you hear about her adventure today?" one asked, obviously tickled by the story. "She is really something."

"What an amazing baby," another nurse said.

The nurses had a Polaroid camera at their disposal, and they used it to take photos so parents who had no babies in their arms could at least carry pictures home. Darlene, the day nurse who'd been nearby when Sarah extubated herself, had taken a moment in the twenty minutes when Sarah was tube-free and asked another nurse to take a picture. In the photograph Darlene holds Sarah, dressed in her yellow gown, perched upright in the isolette, and facing the camera. Sarah's eyes are wide open, her face not happy but not crying either, arms up in the air with fingers spread wide. Someone held a hose that blew humidified oxygen in the direction of Sarah's nose and mouth. That photograph was the first view I'd had of Sarah's face without ET tube and tape in the way, and I just stared at it. There was a cute baby under all the tape. A blue sticky note was attached to the bottom of the photo. On it Darlene had written, "Look, Ma, no tube!"

Until that moment, I hadn't been able to guess at who Sarah might be. Eyes closed. Eyes opened. Eyes scrunched tightly when she was disturbed. That was it. Not only were the physical changes in Sarah so minuscule that I couldn't see them, but whatever personality she might possess was so overwhelmed by her equipment that it never could shine through in a way I could interpret.

The nurses, bless them, saw something in Sarah right from the beginning. They were unabashed in their affection for her and kind in their attention to Jeff and me. I think they felt hopeful about Sarah, because with each day that passed without some disaster occurring, she improved her chances of survival with all systems intact. With experience on their side, they were more optimistic than I was able to be.

Many babies in the unit had physical disabilities they would have to live with forever. I know the staff must have cared for those babies with skill but also with heavy hearts. Sarah, on the other hand, had a chance to do well. She was responding to the high beam of effort aimed at her. Maybe because Jeff was a physician and I a nurse, the nurses could identify with us. They knew if we could have a baby like Sarah, they must be vulnerable as well. Whatever their reasons, the nurses were able to visualize, in a way I could not, that somewhere inside a baby who looked pathetic and emaciated to me, there existed a round-headed butterball. They recognized Sarah's fighting spirit. One nurse tried to explain it to me. She said, "It's as if she's wearing a pair of boxing gloves on her tiny fists, and she's trying her hardest to land her first punch." On the day Sarah extubated herself, I could almost believe the nurse was right.

3 / 2 / 86 Day 49; weight 950 grams: Alert, active, pink; nothing by mouth; weight loss probably due to Lasix dose; intubated on 24% oxygen, 30 breaths per minute. No apnea, bradycardia, chest clear, no murmur, abdomen soft. No further signs of sepsis.

In spite of the obvious progress Sarah was making, her weight gains and losses were measurable only in grams each day. Each ounce represents just under 30 grams, and things moved very slowly. We slogged through March days that seemed as thick as the mud in the local cornfields where the spring thaw was in progress. Sarah's condition was relatively stable, but there was never a day when I felt sure enough to call a friend to say, "Hey! The baby is doing better today! The doctors say she is going to make it!" The only emergencies she experienced were the episodes of apnea and bradycardia that occurred at seemingly random intervals. She was still on the ventilator.

3 / 3 / 86 Day 50; weight 992 grams (up 42 grams): Consider feeding later this week.

3 / 4 / 86 Day 51; weight 964 grams (down 28 grams): Self-extubated this a.m. Reintubated. We will continue to wean from the ventilator. Goal is to reach minimal setting, then hold. Would like to establish some enteral intake before extubating. Assessment and plan discussed with mother.

3 / 5 / 86 Day 52; weight 936 grams (down 28 grams): Start oral feeds, ½ strength breast milk, 1 cc every 3 hours. Watch weight.

3 / 7 / 86 Day 54; weight 964 grams (up 14 grams): Abdomen soft, no masses. Stool heme negative. Stable and appears to be tolerating feedings well. Increase feeds to 3 cc.

3 / 8 / 86 Day 55; 992 grams (up 28 grams): Tolerating feedings well. Working up to good caloric intake.

3 / 9 / 86 Day 56; weight 1005 grams (up 13 grams): 5 bradys on last 2 shifts. Chest X-ray shows endotracheal tube high—tube position adjusted. Reviewed plan with Dad: maintain on ventilator for about 2 weeks and increase feeds. Hopefully to get central venous line out. Use small ET to avoid airway damage.

Maybe Jeff felt confident enough in March to say that Sarah was making progress, but I always thought he was trying to protect me, so I dismissed his opinion as overly optimistic. I continued to live in a state of suspended anxiety tinged with depression. Or maybe it was the other way around.

3 / 12 / 86 Day 59; weight 964 grams (no change for 3 days): Feedings proceeding very well. Can switch to ¾ strength breastmilk at 10 cc / feeding. Exam unchanged from yesterday except murmur audible today.

3 / 14 / 86 Day 61; weight 950 grams (down 15 grams): Continue to increase feeds every 12 hours. Change to full strength at 15 cc. (This will equal 120 cc / kg / d).

3 / 15 / 86 Day 62; weight 978 grams (up 28 grams): Pink, quiet but active at times. No murmur.

My sense of being slowly tortured didn't come from anything bad that happened but because of all the things that didn't. Sarah's weight would go up a few grams, and then, for no explainable reason, it dropped. She was off the vent for a few hours when the tube was dislodged then back on the vent until she was stronger, off the vent again because she'd tugged on the tube, then back on the vent. She was digesting milk but not tolerating very much volume, and the doctors would hold the feedings while they experimented with removing the ET tube. As they tried to wean her from the ventilator, Sarah lost weight because she was expending so much energy with the breathing. I fretted about that. She couldn't afford to lose weight.

3 / 17 / 86 Day 64; weight 1006 grams (up 1 ½ grams): Attending note: Baby is now 64 days of age and quite comfortable being ventilated at a rate of 10, pressures 12 / 3 on room air. Full feedings have nearly been achieved. At this point we can begin to consider extubation at full feeds prior to which we will institute the theophylline. This might come as soon as the end of this week.

On March 19 she gained some weight—I was happy—but later the same day, the lab results showed white blood cells in her urine. My happiness dissolved into worry. Almost every day one problem or another developed. On no day was there enough of what I wanted to see in terms of forward movement.

3 / 19 / 86 Day 66; weight 992 grams (no change): Baby is doing well and should be extubated tonight. There is a urine which was noted to be leukocyte positive; we will repeat urinalysis to look for the absence or presence of white blood cells, particularly given her past history of the candida infection.

During afternoon rounds on March 19, the doctors decided to try a controlled extubation in spite of the white blood cells in her urine.

"What exactly does that mean?" I asked the attending physician. Sarah had been reasonably stable for a few days and weighed just over two pounds.

"A controlled extubation means that removing the tube would be our idea instead of hers," he answered with a hint of a twinkle in his eyes.

To prepare for extubation, the doctors ordered that Sarah receive a dose of intravenous Decadron, a steroid to decrease inflammation and swelling in the trachea. Because the ET tube had been in Sarah's airway for more than two months, its removal was expected to cause a rebound of swelling in the airway. Breathing through a swollen airway was like trying to suck air through a narrow straw. That would be difficult, stressful, and ultimately dangerous, so the doctors wanted to minimize tracheal swelling. Removing the tube also forced Sarah to coordinate a number of physical demands. Her brain needed to signal her lungs to inhale enough times per minute to provide oxygen to her tissues, and her lungs needed to respond with the inhalations as directed. Her body needed to be able to take in enough calories so she could muster the energy to take one breath and another and another. The nurses withheld her feedings on the evening of March 19, as ordered, and administered the Decadron at two a.m. in preparation for extubation at eight o'clock the next morning.

3 / 20 / 86 Day 67; weight 992 grams (no change): Feeding on hold today while being extubated.

And later:

Received Decadron at 2 a.m. Extubated at 8:20 a.m.

I drove to the hospital on the morning of the scheduled procedure with a mixture of hope and dread brewing in my stomach. I didn't know which emotion to trust. When I walked into the NICU at 9:15, I took a minute to orient myself, somehow surprised that the place looked the same as always. All seemed quiet in the blue-white light that had become so familiar. I didn't even see a nurse in Sarah's territory. I moved toward her isolette a little warily, not sure of what I would find. After what seemed like a long walk across the room, I stopped in front of the isolette and tilted my head sideways to get a good look at her.

She lay sleeping on her tummy. She was dressed in a gown and the pink booties, but everything about her seemed different. She looked uncomplicated, almost snuggled into the sheepskin that padded the mattress. No tube came from her mouth. No tape stuck to her skin. Her face was soft and peaceful, sweeter than I had imagined. I had never seen the apples of her cheeks before. The only time I'd seen her without tape and tube was in that Polaroid photo that had been taken a few weeks before, but there was no fullness to her face then. Now she breathed quietly, fifty-five minutes after the extubation. The movement of her back as the air moved in and out of her lungs seemed quiet and absolutely normal.

I didn't want to disturb her, but I had to touch her. I opened the porthole of the isolette without allowing any sound to come from the latch and slipped my hand in, letting it settle on her back like a blanket of feathers.

My time with Sarah that morning was as undisturbed as any I'd had with her. The heart monitor continued its beep . . . beep . . . beep, but that seemed a reassurance rather than an intrusion. The ventilator was pushed a little distance away from Sarah's station and was silent. No lights flashed on its blank face. It stood like a sentry, ready to be activated if called to duty but looking lifeless and abandoned nonetheless. I understood how Luke Skywalker must have felt when the bad guys in Star Wars disabled R2D2. The ventilator was only a machine just as R2D2 was only a robot, but I felt as if it deserved an award for its loyal service.

Nurses came by to peek at Sarah while I sat there. Even they were quieter than usual, not wanting to cause the baby any stress. This was a landmark day, a bend in the road that Sarah had to negotiate, and they were rooting for her. Her breathing and heart rate remained steady through the morning. I left at eleven thirty, feeling as if I needed to tiptoe through the rest of the day and trying not to make any ripples in the air for fear they might come back to disturb my baby.

3 / 20 / 86, continued: Attending note: Baby was extubated at 8:30 this morning and is now comfortable in room air. Stridor which is not audible in the isolette is audible by stethoscope. Based on this we will not feed the child for some 24 hours to insure adequate protection of the airway. Should the child be able to phonate during this time, feedings can then be instituted.

I took little notice of the traffic or the road conditions or the emerging signs of spring as I drove north that day. When I turned into

Lynda's driveway at twelve thirty, it hardly seemed possible I could already be there. I brought Lynda up-to-date on Sarah's status and said hellos and good-byes to the kids while I gathered Willie and his belongings. As soon as we arrived home and took off our coats, I popped him into his high chair for lunch. When he'd swallowed the last of his noodles, he raised his arms in surrender. I lifted him out of his chair and carried him up the stairs and into his room.

While Willie napped, I did laundry, vacuumed floors, and started dinner, but I gave chores as little thought as I had the scenery on the highway. My attention was on this feeling, this hope, this prayer that I carried in my chest: *this* is the day. Or should the emphasis have been, this *is* the day? Whichever it was, through the high-energy afternoon of washing and drying and sweeping and folding and slicing and dicing, my prayer continued over the hours in its various translations and variations in emphasis, Oh, God, *please* let this be the day.

The afternoon passed, but the clock seemed to be wrong every time I looked at it. I wanted to call the unit. I didn't want to call. That is, I only wanted to call if the news was going to be good. If it wasn't going to be good, I wanted to be in the dark for a few more hours. No, I didn't. Yes, I did. I felt as if I were shadow-boxing.

Willie woke around three-thirty per his routine. At four o'clock, he sat in front of *Sesame Street*, and I took the opportunity to call the unit. Pete came to the phone. Right away I could hear there was no lilt in her voice. She sounded somber and almost apologetic.

"She's been having some trouble," she said.

"What kind of trouble?" I asked her.

"Around two o'clock she started having some stridor and then some chest retractions. She had a few bradys, and now she is looking a little dusky around the mouth." Pete paused. Sarah was having respiratory distress. I didn't say anything because I knew what was coming.

"They've decided to reintubate her as soon as they finish afternoon rounds."

The feeling that seeped in with Pete's words was much more familiar than what I had been carrying with me throughout the day. Happiness had floated light and airy in my chest. It expanded my rib cage and allowed my heart more space, and the muscle had been able to beat out a bigger and stronger rhythm. The return of dread was like a brick dropped to the bottom of my stomach. It was as hard and indigestible as it had ever been.

3 / 21 / 86 Day 68; weight 968 grams (down 28 grams, or about 1 oz.): Began having occasional apnea and bradycardia. Clinically—deep retraction with some gasping. Reintubated for clinical condition. Condition improved after intubation.

I was certain with each failure that Sarah was in danger of never being able to breathe without the machine. What would happen if she couldn't come off the ventilator? Would they suddenly say one day, "Sorry, folks, we've done what we can. We have nothing more to offer." Then what would we be faced with? I knew if she did not tolerate breathing without the tube very soon, they would have to take the tube out and surgically perform a tracheotomy. A more permanent tube would be sewn into her neck to take the pressure of the ET tube off her throat and vocal cords. Then what? Raise a child who needed to be on a ventilator for the rest of her life? A child who would have no voice? At what point would they make that decision?

What I needed was for one of the doctors to take me by the shoulders, look me square in the eye, and say, "Susan, we see X babies like Sarah each year. She is smaller than most, but she has made good progress. It will probably take a few tries before she can get off the machine, but we are not worried. Everything else looks good, and she will do it. Be patient. She just needs some time." But no one did that, either because they really didn't know what she was capable of or because they had no idea how desperate I felt each time they said, "We replaced the tube today." The sentence sounded so benign, but I knew what it meant. I had been there on an evening when Sarah was having trouble with the placement with her tube and had to be re-intubated.

The staff had been concerned about ventilator pressures indicating Sarah's tube was out of place. A doctor and two nurses gathered around Sarah's isolette and positioned themselves to remove the tube in Sarah's mouth and replace it with another. I'd quietly stepped out of the way while the caregivers moved with quiet purpose. One nurse helped position Sarah's neck. The doctor stood at Sarah's head, his face looking down at hers, his body bent forward. His hands held a metallic tongue blade that illuminated the pathway into Sarah's narrow throat, and he worked it to pry Sarah's lips apart. When her mouth opened—but not willingly like a baby robin's would if it anticipated the bugs that its mother carried—I could see the instrument press deeply back on Sarah's tongue. She gagged, trying to escape the hands and the discomfort of the position, the threat of it. Her entire body wiggled, and the nurses held her arms and legs still. The doctor picked up a new plastic tube from the sterile field set up on a tray beside him and brought the tip of it to Sarah's face. The disproportionately large gloved hands slipped the tube into the baby's mouth and down her throat once—nope. He pulled it out, tried again—and then I heard his voice, "There we go," and he sounded relieved. One nurse taped the endotracheal tube to Sarah's face while the other attached Sarah's tube to the one that led to the ventilator. The muted whoosh of the mechanical breathing re-started. Sarah lay silent, breathing on command, tethered once again. When the team dispersed, I stepped up to the isolette, opened the porthole, and covered her body with my hand. She lay still, defeated, and I felt helpless, unable to protect her from anything. The doctors and nurses were the good guys, after all. Sarah still couldn't manufacture tears, but mine made up for hers.

3 / 25 / 86 Day 72; weight 992 grams (up 28 grams): Sarah has not shown consistent weight gain; accordingly we are advancing feeds and after 7 days of consecutive weight gain, will attempt extubation again. During this time, hopefully, edema from the previous 3.0 tube will have decreased slightly given the presence of the 2.5 tube now.

Though I didn't want to see it, the intubation scene replayed in my head each time a nurse or a doctor matter-of-factly reported to me after an extubation, "We had to reintubate the baby." If I tried to erase the vision by closing my eyes, the rerun only became more vivid and more awful.

After the failed attempt at removing the tube on March 20, the doctors said Sarah would have to gain weight for seven consecutive days before they would try to remove it again. That meant there was no hope that she would come off the vent for at least a week, which seemed a far stretch down a long road, especially when, as the days of that week went by, she did not gain in any kind of steady pattern. On March 22 she weighed 978 grams (two pounds and two-and-one-half ounces.) On the twenty-third she dropped to 964 grams, and the next day she stayed at that same weight. On the twenty-fifth she jumped to 992 grams, and on the twenty-sixth another gain to 1021 grams, but on the twenty-seventh and the twenty-eighth her weight stayed at 1021 grams. We were still at square one with zero consecutive days of weight gain. I chafed. I couldn't stand the wait.

Apparently, Sarah was also growing impatient with the pace because sometime in the early morning hours of March 28 she once again took matters into her own hands. Though she hadn't gained weight as required and no controlled extubation was scheduled, the ET tube somehow became dislodged.

On those occasions when she extubated herself, she did not actually pull the tube all the way out of her mouth. That would have required the peeling of intricately arranged strips of white tape from her face or from the tube and more strength and sense of purpose than she possessed. However, while it might look as if Sarah were sleeping, her hand would rest on the length of tube where it lay on the sheets as a child might hold the stick of a lollipop while she sucked on it. Sarah's fingers would fiddle with the plastic or she'd squirm enough so eventually the tube would be wiggled out of the proper position in her trachea. The ventilator alarmed when it detected a change of pressure in the air delivered to her lungs. Then a doctor or the NICU clinical nurse specialist would have to pull the tube out and insert a new one.

When Sarah extubated herself in the middle of the night of March 28, the doctor working that shift decided to give Sarah another chance to breathe on her own. He instructed the staff to watch her for a few hours rather than try to re-intubate right away. Sarah breathed humidified air under her own power all that night.

3 / 28 / 86 Day 75; weight 1021 grams (no change): Self-extubated last night. Has been stable since on room air. Stridor audible with stethoscope but seems comfortable. No racemic epinephrine was required. Leave on room air if tolerated.

That was all there was to it. No fanfare. No IV Decadron. No withheld feedings. She simply continued to prove on that day, one breath after another, one hour after another, that she could breathe on her own.

3 / 29 / 86 Day 76; weight 1021 grams (no change): Taking 12 cc every 2 hours ½ strength breast milk and ½ strength 24 calorie formula. Abdomen full but soft—minimal residuals. No spitting. Room air. Apnea and brady X1. Self-corrected.

I came in on Saturday morning to find her in her isolette, untaped and untubed. Watching her breathe on her own made me think of a little sprite I had seen skating on Barton Cove one Sunday that winter when the sun had been warm and the ice populated with colorful groups of fisherman. Dogs skittered around their owners and one another, their four feet even less sure on the ice than the humans' two. Kids pulled each other on saucers or skated on the river's glassy surface. The little girl couldn't have been more than five years old. She had spent the afternoon on her skates, wobbling around a man I presumed to be her father while he drilled holes in the ice and set his lines. Both of the child's ankles were collapsed in her skates, and she teetered on the outside blade edges in a way that made my own ankles hurt with the memory. When I happened to walk through the kitchen every now and again, my eye would invariably be drawn outside to the would-be skater, her lack of balance so obvious next to the other upright humans who stood in their rubber-soled boots. More than once I saw the fluorescent pink arms of her jacket flail when her skates left the ice and she sat down hard. She got up again. I saw it a few times, but I'm sure it had been happening all afternoon.

Finally, for no good reason I could discern, the little girl stuck out a skate and it did something different. It glided on the ice. Then she performed the same trick with the other skate. One foot followed another until she was moving across the ice. I had parked Willie on the countertop where he folded his legs Indian-style and watched with me although his eyes were on the dogs. The little girl remained upright, each foot wobbling through an abbreviated glide.

4 / 1 / 86 Day 79; weight 1077 grams: Attending note:. History reviewed. Alert, active, pink. Chest clear, heart rate regular, no murmur. Abdomen soft. Extremities warm. Tone: movements symmetric. Assessment: growing premature. Talked to Mom. Plan: transfer to Greenfield at 1500 grams (3 pounds 2 ounces).

As March came to an end, little Sarah finally performed her own version of the ice skater's dance forty miles away from the scene I'd watched from my kitchen window. She kept doing it just like the little Barton Cove skater. Air in. Air out. Fall down. Get help. Get up. Hold on. Let go. Air in. Air out. She was wobbly, but she breathed on her own and kept going, one inspired moment after another.

BOTTLE VS. BREAST: ROUND ONE

When Sarah was finally extubated for good, I gave in to worries about sight, hearing, and brain function. The doctors had a weight goal, but no one named a date for when she would come home. I was in danger of turning into one of the parents who sat complaining for hours in the waiting area. Usually I avoided hanging out in the parents' room, first because I wanted to spend every minute with Sarah, and later because I did not want to get caught up in the negativity of the families who sat there. I had enough floating around in my own head without heaping the unhappiness of the other parents on top of mine.

Even with the growing squeak of my own complaints, I found it surprising to overhear how dissatisfied the babies' families were. Frightened and unable to protect their children from disease or disaster, the parents who sat in the waiting room had nowhere to put their anger, upset, and guilt but on the doctors and nurses. I found it disturbing to overhear their misinterpretation or misunderstanding of medical information. I had to bite my tongue to keep from saying, "No, no, no! You've got it all wrong!"

Eventually even I became dissatisfied with the doctors who, I thought, were not paying enough attention to my baby now that she was less critical than others in the unit. They seemed unconcerned about her lack of steady weight gain and satisfied with her plodding progress. I became another of the NICU parents who considered herself an authority, if not in neonatology, at least in the care of her own child. As far as I was concerned, the doctors were being too cautious with Sarah's feedings.

"All she needs to do is gain some weight," was the daily pronouncement at Sarah's bedside. The doctors were actually beginning to talk about Sarah's future. The plan was for her to be transferred to Franklin Medical Center when she reached three pounds and two ounces. Yet she remained stuck at two pounds and two ounces for two days. Three days. Four. How could she gain weight if they didn't increase the amount of her feedings? I suspected that Sarah was being followed primarily by less experienced residents and not the attending neonatologists. The specialists saw Sarah on rounds each day, I knew, but I could see their time was consumed by the newborn babies who were in crisis. The doctors ordered 30 cc per feeding, and when she tolerated that, they increased the feeding by only two cc. One ounce every two hours. How can she grow on that? I wondered. How will she ever get out of here?

I should have been happier as March turned into April. Sarah was obviously making progress. There were many unknowns, but the trend was positive. I could finally believe she would come home one day. A long-squelched worry, however, turned to a new obsession, and it rose to the top of my list of things to be anxious about. Sarah was not breast-feeding.

When Sarah finally looked as though she would survive, I hung my hat on a long-submerged hope. Breast-feeding seemed to be the one normal baby function she still could experience. The upbeat voice of the La Leche nurse haunted me. I had spent the winter sitting on my cold bathroom floor with the electric machine. I had continued to pump my breasts three to four times a day from January into April in the hope that, if Sarah lived, she would eventually nurse. The pump nurse had been unequivocal about it. The books about premature babies said it was possible. The La Leche woman on the phone said, "Oh, definitely, this can work. And breast milk is best for the baby." The nurses in the NICU said, "Yes, well, it's possible," but their eyes did not meet mine when they said so. While I held on to the possibilities, the nurses introduced Sarah to her first oral feedings. My yearning to nurse the baby gnawed at me as each day passed. Sarah took milk first by tube and then by bottle but not by breast.

"She took a bottle this morning," a nurse told me one day in April. She sounded pleased. "Ten cc. And she kept it down nicely."

"She did?" I said. My smile played for her as expected, but I could feel how tightly it spread across my face.

Since the authorities said preemies could breast-feed, I assumed I could nurse her from her first feedings. I hadn't considered the reality of how many feedings I could actually be present for in a day and how many other times in a twenty-four-hour day she would need to drink from a bottle. She was like a hummingbird, needing small, frequent feedings every two hours at the minimum. I calculated. That was twelve feedings a day, and I could be there for how many? One, maybe two, if I went back in the evening.

Breast-feeding is all I have left with this baby, I thought. It was the only part of her infancy that I could possibly salvage. Breast-feeding was the last concrete, physical connection I would have with Sarah, and I was certain she would be our last child. I harbored the hope that breast-feeding would work out and carried my hope in a bubble protected from all the facts recorded on the day sheet that hung on a clipboard at the end of her isolette.

Nurses weighed and measured every drop of liquid that went into Sarah's body and every one that came out, including their calculations for insensible loss. I wondered, how can they know how many calories she takes in if she nurses?

Two days after Sarah extubated herself, she continued to do well breathing on her own. I sat in a rocking chair while Darlene prepared Sarah for the complicated process of coming out of her isolette. This was the day I would try to breast-feed Sarah. Darlene bundled the baby in a blanket and stretched a stocking cap over her head. Then she handed the baby to me.

I settled Sarah into a position that should have been familiar to both of us but instead made me feel all thumbs. I fumbled under my shirt, not feeling the letdown of milk I remembered from days with Willie but instead a letdown of emotion at the bright lights, the monitors, the open room, and the lack of privacy. I had anticipated a sweet and solemn moment to spend with my baby. Instead, I felt it was yet another side show under the big top of the complicated, technical intensive care circus.

I positioned Sarah's face towards my body and rubbed my nipple against her cheek. She turned instinctively, opening her mouth into a small O, and I felt a small surge of confidence.

Nursing is natural, I assured myself. Look at how she automatically moves her face towards my breast. Sarah tugged at my nipple with some curiosity, and I watched her cheeks hollow as she tried out what her instincts told her to do. Then, as suddenly as she had moved towards the suckling, she stopped and turned her face away from me. I placed my hand under my breast, squeezed from the base down to my thumb and index finger at the nipple, and urged milk to appear. A few white droplets obliged, but Sarah continued to face away from me.

"Okay," I said, "we can switch if you like it better the other way." I moved her to my other arm and repositioned her. I rocked her and crooned, "Come on, Sweetie Pie. Come on. This is good. Have some milk." She struggled and turned her head away. She made her opinion clear. She wanted none of this. I felt embarrassed, suddenly ashamed of the exposure. I pulled my shirt back into some order, rocked back and forth in the chair, and tried not to panic.

"Darlene?" I called to her. She stood at the nurses' station and shuffled papers, probably trying not to hover.

She came to me and gently chided as she picked Sarah up and placed her back in the isolette.

"What are you up to, huh?" She continued talking as she unbundled Sarah from the blanket, settled her on the sheepskin, and reattached monitor lines. "You have to eat so that you can grow big and get out of here. You need to have your morning snack. Now what are we going to do?" She reattached the lines to the cardiac monitor and turned the machine on.

Sarah lay still, her eyes tightly closed. No comment.

As each day passed, she took more from the preemie bottles the nurses offered her. An ounce of liquid is equal to thirty cc. Her bottle held two ounces. She started by taking ten cc at a time, and if she digested that (the nurse would measure two hours after the feeding by slipping a tube in through her nose and into her stomach and withdrawing any remaining liquid), she would get the same amount for the next feeding. If she had milk left in her stomach, even just two cc, the nurse would withhold the next scheduled feeding. Doctors' orders. They were still concerned that liquids left in her stomach after one or two hours might indicate her intestines were not functioning properly. If she digested her feedings well for two consecutive days, the doctors would order an increase in her feeding by a few cc.

She crawled forward by droplets, and very few of them came from me. In my heart, I kept postponing the time when I believed it would be critical for Sarah to begin nursing. The thoughts started to take form in March: I will breast-feed her as soon as she can start taking oral liquids. I don't want her to get used to a bottle, so I will come as often as I can to feed her. I ignored the lecture I used to give my prenatal patients: "If you are planning to nurse, don't give the baby any bottles for the first month. She needs to get used to feeding from the breast. It is harder work for the baby, and if she gets used to the different smell and easy flow of the formula through the artificial nipple, she will refuse to feed from the breast." I began to create a theory I could live with. Maybe preemies didn't have the same requirements imprinted on their brains in the way full-term babies do. I decided to defer the serious feeding lessons until Sarah moved closer to home. Breast-feeding will be easier when she gets to the hospital in Greenfield, I rationalized. We'll have more time together then.

I developed a routine when I visited Sarah. I would pick her up at feeding time and we'd settle into a rocking chair. First, I would offer her the breast. When she sniffed around for a bit and decided she wasn't interested, I squelched the sadness that threatened to overwhelm me and reached for a bottle that had been prepared by the nurse. Sarah took the pliant rubber nipple into her mouth and sucked, eyes closed. I watched the level of the white liquid recede slowly until the bottle was empty. As one April visit followed another, I fed and then rocked the little bit of who she was—she still weighed just a touch over two pounds—until she dropped into a satisfied sleep. After placing her back in the isolette, I drove home, sat with the breast pump for ten minutes, froze the decreasing quantities of milk I produced, and refused to acknowledge the persistent questions, what is the point of torturing yourself, Susan? Why do you bother?

ON BECOMING A GROWER

Once Sarah was extubated and breathing competently on her own, there was no need for the moment-to-moment nursing care she had required. There came a day in April when I walked into the unit, and she wasn't there.

"She's moved next door," a nurse said, pointing to the room I could see through the window that formed one wall of the NICU. The intermediate unit was adjacent to the NICU and a step down in intensity. The nursing staff still watched patients closely, but the babies in intermediate care were not on ventilators. They were less sick, and the baby-to-nurse ratio was higher.

Moving Sarah had been a matter of rolling the isolette a few yards across one room and into the adjoining room, no different than if I'd carried her from my kitchen to the living room, but the fact that she had been moved out of the NICU was rather a shock. Her coming off the ventilator successfully had been such an overriding goal that my thinking hadn't moved on to what would happen after she accomplished that. The next step in the process should have been obvious: extubation meant Sarah didn't need to be in the NICU. When I thought about it, I hadn't seen a baby in the NICU who was not on a ventilator. It did make sense. Free of the ventilator, finished with antibiotics, feeding from a bottle, she was less needy.

I was not with Sarah when she moved through the door from one room to the next, and I felt wistful about missing that transition. Although the physical distance she had traveled was negligible, it was a monumental step for her to move out of the NICU. It felt weird for the staff to have moved her without telling me it was going to happen. Or maybe they had said it was coming, and I didn't hear or chose to ignore the possibility.

I'm her mother. I should have been there, I thought.

Of course I didn't need to be there, but I could not shed my sense of responsibility for the baby despite the fact that I had never been responsible for her care. Neither could I shake the sense of loss that came out of her premature separation from me. Every separation reverberated with that feeling. I hated that her life moved forward for twenty-three hours each day without my being there to watch or be a part of it. Mothers and babies have to open up the space between them at some time. Babies spend their first year learning they are separate from their mothers. What I hadn't thought about was the second part of the equation. In the first year, a mother also needs to learn her baby is no longer part of her. I wasn't ready to hear that message.

When Sarah moved to be with the other growers, she left nurses who had been dedicated to her since January. In those months I had developed relationships with those nurses. I had spent many hours hovering with David, Lauren, Pete, Denise, and Jackie in the zone that surrounded Sarah. I had spoken with them on the phone every day. We all shared the same baby. Sarah's physicians would be the same in intermediate care, so they would still be in the picture. But I would miss the nurses, not so much as individuals, perhaps, but as a solid unit I had come to trust. Our interactions had not been overly sentimental—Sarah was their patient and their duty was to her. But I thought of them as I would a line of police in uniform or firefighters dressed in all of their gear. In my mind the nurses stood shoulder to shoulder in their blue and green scrubs and allowed nothing to get by the zone of safety they created around my baby. They would be impossible to replace.

Unbeknownst to me, however, Sarah's arrival in the intermediate unit had been greatly anticipated. Because she had earned a reputation as a fighter, Sarah had also engaged the special interest of the intermediate care nurses. They had been looking through the window, following her progress, watching and waiting for her to come through their door. There had been some good-natured sparring over who would be Sarah's primary nurse. Finally, I could see enough of a baby to know why.

Without the endotracheal tube, Sarah had turned into a petite Munchkin of a baby. As she began tolerating fats in her intravenous line and then high calorie formula through the feeding tube, the first weight she gained was in her cheeks. The sight of that face made me smile. It seemed as if overnight she developed chipmunk cheeks, prominent little bulges that pouched out as if she were storing something good for later in the day. Apparently it was a normal pattern of early fat distribution in preemies, not surprising to the doctors and nurses but amusing to Jeff and me. The cheeks gave her the look of instant health.

Even with her first layer of facial fat, the rest of Sarah's body remained skeletal. The prime directive remained clear: she needed to gain weight. In the intermediate unit, the babies were not all as tiny as she was, and they hadn't necessarily started in the NICU. Some were bigger, older, and recovering from their complicated births. One was on feedings administered through a tube that had been permanently sewn into his stomach. He'd had most of his intestine surgically removed due to the devastating intestinal condition NEC, one complication Sarah had avoided. One baby was still very small and not growing. He needed oxygen and tube feedings because his lungs were underdeveloped at birth. Another baby had a genetic disorder that made feeding difficult. He wouldn't live much longer, the nurse told me as she changed his position on the mattress.

A few days after Sarah moved to her new home, I noticed a new patient admission in the space across from hers. While Sarah personified the diminutive as she slept quietly on her tummy, the new baby in blue blankets lay florid and logy on his back as if he had just come from the feast of Dionysus. Pudgy was a kind but inadequate description for this baby, who had been born the previous night. His face was so fat he could hardly open his eyes. This baby was Winston Churchill to Sarah's Audrey Hepburn. If Sarah and the boy baby had been placed on opposite ends of a seesaw, it would have taken almost five Sarahs to counterweight the big boy.

I allowed myself a smile at Winston's expense and then looked at the nurse who was about to prick the baby's heel for a blood sample.

"Diabetic?" I asked.

The nurse nodded.

The baby's mother must have had poorly controlled diabetes during her pregnancy. Overloaded with sugar during the months in utero, he had grown fat from storing all of the extra fuel he couldn't use. He was in the unit because he needed to be watched closely. Once he was separated from his mother's placenta, his own blood sugars would plunge as his liver and pancreas tried to regulate the glucose levels in his blood.

His stay in the unit was brief. Two days after I'd first seen the chubby baby, his spot in the unit was empty. His blood sugars had stabilized, and his mother had taken her prizefighter home.

Sarah finished her last course of antibiotics at the end of March. In April, her only medicines were a liquid vitamin and theophylline to stimulate her breathing. For the first time she was able to take all of her nutrition by mouth, and she no longer needed an IV. Some days I tried nursing her, and some days I didn't feel up to the challenge. Once again, I promised myself we would start in a few weeks when she was transferred to the hospital near our home.

Time dragged. When Jeff and I lived in central Washington, apple orchards exploded with blossoms on April first. On my drive to the Community Health Center I passed acres of trees enveloped in pink clouds. When we lived in New Haven, April brought warm rains and early forsythia. But in Gill, where Massachusetts meets Vermont, the skies of early spring were gray more often than not, and the sun was never as warm as I thought it should be. I turned thirty-two on the tenth of April, and snowflakes blew sideways across my windshield as I drove to the hospital.

On too many of those April days, the scale showed no change in Sarah's weight, or she would gain and lose the same few grams. The doctors remained conservative with her feedings, increasing them not by ounces but by drops. It was all I could do not to have a temper tantrum à la Willie and yell, "Feed her more."

One day seemed to blend into the next, but gradually changes did happen. Sarah's chipmunk cheeks deflated and became less prominent as the fat distributed evenly over her body. Her head was still flattened on the sides, her face was long and narrow, and she spent most of her time sleeping. When she opened her eyes, however, she looked out on her world with indisputable alertness. She developed some substance to her arms and legs. Her skin looked pliable and elastic as her limbs softened and took shape. The bright red birthmark still sat like a custom-fitted ruby above her forehead but looked smaller as her head and body grew.

In spite of the fits and starts in her weight gain pattern, by the third week of April Sarah finally reached the milestone we were waiting for. On the day she reached three pounds, the doctors called our pediatrician in Greenfield and made arrangements for her to be transferred to the hospital closer to home. She could leave Baystate when she reached three pounds and two ounces.

On the evening before Sarah was due to be transferred to the hospital in Greenfield, I scrubbed at the hospital sink, dressed in a gown, and walked into the intermediate care area to find Sarah's spot taken up by a stranger. I wasn't exactly alarmed, but the adrenaline response at the disappearance of my child was automatic, just as it would be if I had been playing in the park with Willie and he'd suddenly disappeared. A nurse looked up from tube-feeding a baby and said apologetically, "We had to move her this afternoon. She's in the growers' room."

Sarah had been transferred to the next step-down unit. I hadn't known there was another level of care. It was for babies who needed only to gain weight before they could go home. Lots of preemies never needed the NICU. They were born early or small and just needed to feed and grow before they were discharged. Usually they left the hospital when they reached five pounds. From the window I could see row upon row of isolettes. Can't they keep her in the intermediate unit for one more night? I thought, feeling abandoned. The new place seemed so impersonal. I didn't know anyone there.

I walked into the room and waited. A woman in scrubs sat feeding a baby and talking to another woman who appeared to be a hospital employee but not a nurse. A housekeeper, perhaps. The nurse had to know I was standing there but did not move her head or even her eyes to acknowledge my presence. I waited. She finished her thought and went on to the next one. Finally she looked at me, and I introduced myself. I asked where Sarah was. She didn't smile or greet me but just pointed to the farthest corner of the room. Do you have any idea who my baby is? I wanted to ask her. Do you know what she has been through? And you have her parked way out there? I flashed to my grading system, which had been dormant for a while, and gave the woman an *F*.

This unit was in the business of mass-feeding babies. I remembered a room like it from a night at Yale-New Haven when I was pulled from a slow shift at the pediatric ICU to help out in the neonatal unit. Since I didn't know what to do with babies that small, they put me in the feeding room where I wouldn't be a danger to anyone. I picked up a baby, weighed it, fed it from a bottle until it tired, then inserted a nasogastric tube through one little nostril and let the rest of the prescribed feeding drain in by gravity from a big syringe. I changed the diaper and moved on to the next baby. Nearly two dozen babies later, I was happy to go back to my unit. It was hard to see each baby as anyone's little precious on that shift, and now Sarah was a part of a similar production line.

It was time for Sarah to move on. I wondered if there was a reasoned plan to this step system. Perhaps the care was supposed to get increasingly impersonal in order to wean parents like me from the NICU. Seeing how little attention Sarah would get if she stayed at the big hospital I felt no qualms about moving her to Franklin Medical Center. I had been concerned the nurses at our little community hospital might not be able to handle Sarah's care: her feeding requirements, medicines, and occasional episodes of apnea. But Jeff had confidence in his hospital and no worries at all about the move. A few days earlier I'd met with Jill, the head nurse at Franklin Medical Center's nursery. She had once been a NICU nurse at Baystate. Jill listened attentively to all I said and asked questions that proved she knew exactly what she was talking about. She exuded a quiet competence, and she certainly did not seem concerned about her staff's ability to meet Sarah's needs.

Once I found Sarah in her isolette and assured myself she was okay, I hiked back to the nurse to find out if I could feed Sarah.

"No, she was just fed," said the nurse. Tough luck. As I walked back to Sarah, it occurred to me I needed a plastic flower to hang on the isolette so I could find her the next day. Then I remembered I'd never have to find her there again.

On Monday, April 28, Mercy Ambulance pulled up to the back door of Baystate Medical Center to reverse the trip the unborn Sarah had taken in January. Sarah's due date had been April 24. The day was as sunny as the day of her winter arrival had been, but instead of glittering with a January freeze, the air was warm and the fields between Springfield and Greenfield stretched out in bright green carpets.

I waited at home for the phone call saying Sarah had landed in Greenfield. Jeff later told me an entourage waited at Franklin Medical Center for the much-anticipated baby. He said Sarah exhibited her best avoidance behavior by ignoring her admirers with a frowning face and eyes clamped shut. Once in the hospital's newborn nursery, she was placed in a warm isolette.

By the time I drove the four short miles from home, Sarah was settled in her new place. When I walked in, I saw Jill bent over the new admission. Jill had de-mummified Sarah. The blankets she'd been wrapped in for the trip from Baystate lay in a heap on the mattress, and Jill was listening with a tiny stethoscope to Sarah's heart and lungs. When she finished, she re-wrapped Sarah's chest with the strap from the apnea monitor. Then she untangled the wires from the chest strap and plugged them into the machine. The paperwork on Sarah's clipboard said she weighed three pounds and two ounces.

I looked around the nursery. I felt both excited and nervous about this change, and I needed to adjust to the quiet. No alarms. No flashing lights. A few cribs held infants wrapped in pink or blue, and another nurse worked over a baby at the other end of the room. A gray-haired man and woman stood with a small child at the viewing window and pointed to a baby swaddled in blue. The adults wore big, wide smiles. I felt one growing on my own face.

I turned back to my baby. Jill left a porthole open for me. I reached in to touch Sarah. Her eyes were closed. The apnea monitor lights flashed green each time she took a breath.

Green for go, I thought. Go, Baby, go.

HOMECOMING

Sarah's transition to our local hospital was smooth. Being Jeff's daughter gave her VIP status, and she was officially admitted as Sarah Blomstedt. The nurses dressed Sarah in her gowns and booties and fussed over her in a sweet combination of the professional and personal. It seemed as if in the transfer from Springfield she'd shed the trauma of her prematurity and suddenly was the baby I'd been waiting for. Her big eyes set in the small face were magnetic. That look, plus her connection to the greater hospital family, guaranteed a parade of visitors at the nursery window.

I was relieved because I was finally able to spend more time with Sarah. I actually took notice of the sunny days and felt cheerful when I woke in the morning, confident about how I would find Sarah, hopeful about what the day would bring. I felt better knowing Jeff would check on her first thing when he went to work. I went to the hospital later in the morning while Willie was at Lynda's and then again in the evening after Jeff came home.

Sometimes Willie and I visited Sarah together in the afternoon. Those visits were frustrating, though, because I wanted to nurse Sarah on my visits. In general, breast-feeding was not going as well as I'd hoped, but I couldn't even try when I had Willie with me. I brought him so he would become accustomed to the idea there would soon be a new person in our house. In Willie's mind, Sarah had probably been nothing more than a reason for me to be leaving him, as in, "Mommy is going to see Sarah for a little while." Now that she'd moved to Greenfield, Sarah had become real. When I took Willie to the nursery, I would lift him high enough to see into the isolette. I explained who the baby was each time, and he looked at her with a grave expression.

"Hmmmm," he appeared to be thinking as he pressed on his lower lip with a long index finger. Then he would wriggle to get down, and the visit was over.

Sarah left her unfinished look at Baystate. The gradual weight gain showed on her face and in her arms and legs. Her skin finally seemed to fit. Her face and head were well-proportioned to the rest of her body. Someone who didn't know she was a preemie would probably not even notice the elongated shape of her head. She looked like a perfect baby in miniature. She was often awake when I went to see her, and her eyes were dark and seemed very knowing for her size. It made her aura even more compelling because, at three pounds and change, she was smaller than an average newborn yet had the alert look of a baby who had seen a bit of the world. When I arrived at the nursery each day, I couldn't wait to hold her. As soon as I checked in with the nurses, I opened the front of the isolette. I stretched a cap over her head, wrapped the rest of her in a blanket, and swept her out of her box. We sat together and rocked for as long as I could stay. Even if it wasn't feeding time, I offered her the chance to nurse, but she didn't suckle for very long. I was so happy to have her that I couldn't take her rejection seriously. I knew when we had more time and more privacy at home, we could work it out. Pushing away the worry, I would feel the slight weight of her in my arms and wonder how she had survived the winter. I shook my head more than once at the idea that this baby's story might actually have a happy ending.

I should have been satisfied just to have Sarah in Greenfield. But once I got over the initial happiness of having her in town, I finally admitted to my most secret self that I would not feel complete until I had her at home. Nothing else would do. Even though just four miles separated us and her dad could visit her any number of times while he worked, I felt as if I couldn't see her enough. I felt I didn't have enough quiet time to try nursing her. The day was still chopped up between running Willie to Lynda's and spending snatches of time with Sarah. She lived at the hospital and was not a full-fledged member of our family. Jeff and I passed each other on the way in and out of the house as we went to retrieve one child or to visit the other. I was always missing somebody. It had been four months since I had gone to bed at night with the feeling that my entire family was tucked in and accounted for. In the days and weeks and months that had passed since January 12, I had not once felt whole.

Our pediatrician said Sarah should probably stay in the nursery until she weighed five pounds. I was okay with that for about a week and then stopped to count on my fingers. If she gained one half ounce per day as she had been doing, that would add up to . . . oh, way longer than I could stand. Almost two months, and that was if she gained every single day. When she had been at Franklin for a little over two weeks, she reached three pounds and twelve ounces. Her care was routine, and she was stable, feeding well from a bottle and producing wet diapers just as she should. In her feedings, she received drops of various vitamins, and the other medication they gave her was caffeine, of all things, to stimulate her breathing. I remembered how, when I'd been nursing Willie, I had agonized over every drop of caffeine I might drink, over every herb and spice and ounce of tomato sauce I ingested, and I blamed any burp or cry that Willie produced on something I had eaten. Sarah was taking a hit of caffeine every four hours.

By mid-May, spring was in full bloom, and I was antsy. I wanted her to come home. After returning from the hospital one evening, I said to Jeff, "Don't you think we can take care of her at home?"

He looked at me and said, "I don't see why not."

The next morning, I talked to Sarah's doctor when he came into the nursery.

"Hugh," I said. "I think we can do this at home. She is healthy now. Her breathing is good. She has no infections. Her diapers are wet. She is tolerating the breast milk / formula mix from a bottle, and I can feed her on whatever schedule she needs. Maybe I can even get her to breast-feed at home. I can mix her medicines, and she isn't even getting very many. She has the apnea monitor and has hardly had a spell in the three weeks that she's been here. We can even rent an isolette if she still needs to stay in a warm environment." I stopped for a breath. I had to restrain myself from dropping down to my knees and grabbing at his pants legs as I begged. I hounded the poor man until he held up his hands in surrender.

"Well," he said, drawing it out, "usually we wait until the baby weighs five pounds." I groaned. "But, she does seem to be pretty stable."

I brightened.

"I think we can let her go when she reaches four pounds."

I threw my arms around him. Finally, a reachable goal was in sight. At the rate she was gaining, she would weigh four pounds by the end of the week.

After Hugh left the unit, I slipped my hand into the isolette to rub Sarah's back. I could still count her ribs beneath my fingers but also sensed the light padding that now covered her bones. I couldn't stop smiling as I watched her sleep.

In order to ease Sarah's transition from hospital to home, Jeff said he would take Willie out of the picture for the weekend if that would make things better for me. I don't remember whose idea that was, but Jeff probably would have agreed to any plan to placate me. After four months of living with a woman who had just barely held herself together, he was bent like a pretzel trying to accommodate my needs. Jeff decided he and Willie would drive to Pennsylvania to visit Jeff's parents and then would bring Muz back to spend a week with us. That would give me two days alone with Sarah and allow me to adjust to her schedule and start nursing her without having a curious toddler at my knees.

In the late afternoon of May 16, I stood watching as Jeff and Willie disappeared from our driveway in the red station wagon. The right side of our drive was bordered with an outcropping of gray rock, but just that day the fuzzy moss on the rock had been transformed into a green carpet. I knew by the time Jeff returned with Muz and Will, thousands of tiny flowers would burst open, and the rocks would disappear under a cloud of pink. I stood with that image for a few minutes in the afternoon sun and then turned and walked into the house. The first thing I noticed was the quiet. Then I was faced with the domestic scene. I'd made a brown-bag lunch for Jeff and Willie, and the fixings still littered the counter. Willie's toys lay scattered on the floor. I grabbed a laundry basket and started picking up.

I spent the next hours organizing the house and gathering newspapers from countertops and stray trucks from under chairs. I wondered how I could have been so selfish, sending poor Jeff on a six-hour car trip with Willie. I went to the grocery store to stock up for the coming week, and when I returned home, the sun was just setting. It seemed to hang in the air for a long while on that May evening as I prepared for Sarah's homecoming.

Saturday, May 17, 1986 dawned sunny and clear, a quintessential New England spring day. I didn't know quite when to leave for the hospital. I could pick her up any time. I didn't want to get there too soon, interrupting the staff at report and the early obligations of their shift. I didn't want to look overly anxious, like someone arriving at a party too early. So, with time on my hands and nothing else to do, I stood at the kitchen counter and stared at the front page of the newspaper. After taking a few sips of my second cup of coffee, I dumped the rest. I couldn't wait any longer. At eight forty-five I opened the door of the little blue Honda and climbed in.

I settled into the car with a sense of quiet excitement. I remembered what it had felt like to drive with Willie when he was new, how conscientious I had suddenly become when this little person appeared in my car where he lay buckled into his seat and sucking on his fist. That feeling was back as I drove to the Franklin Medical Center, the sense that I needed to drive very carefully to get there. It was the kind of spring day I had imagined for Sarah's birth with rhododendrons in full bloom as I drove into Greenfield.

When I walked into the nursery, the pediatrician who was covering for the weekend was bent over Sarah's isolette. Hugh was not at the hospital. He and I had talked the day before about the plan for taking care of Sarah at home, and he told me to bring Sarah to his office in a week. The pediatrician turned his head, stethoscope in his ears, to bid me a good morning. When he was satisfied with his patient's heartbeat, lung sounds, the softness of her belly, the color in her cheeks, and the normal temperature recorded on the clipboard, he sat at the desk and wrote the final note of Sarah's hospitalization. As the doctor left the nursery, he wished me luck.

The nursery seemed quiet that morning as if everyone, even new babies, had taken the weekend off. I saw only one nurse, whom I hadn't met before. She was working at the isolette and talking to Sarah as if they were old friends. I set down the diaper bag I had carried in with me and pawed through it to find the outfit I'd brought for Sarah's departure from the hospital. It seemed important to pick the right outfit as if it were a bride's trousseau and had to be carefully chosen. Sarah had sort of outgrown the nightgowns my mother had made for her, not in size so much as in maturity. She was no longer going to be a patient and didn't need those little flannel gowns, so for the occasion I decided on a real, store-bought preemie outfit for her to wear. Our neighbors gave it to me as a homecoming present for Sarah, and when I pulled it out of its box, I realized I'd never seen such small baby clothing. I looked for the tag at the back of the neck where the size was usually printed. "Preemie," it said, "to six pounds."

The nurse asked if she could dress Sarah. Though I wanted to scoop the baby up and run away with her, I smiled and said with all the generosity I could muster, "Of course." While the nurse fussed over Sarah, I looked through the pile of "Welcome Baby" freebies the nurse pointed to on a shelf in the corner of the room. As I placed the gifts in a shopping bag decorated with chicks, ducks, and the prominent logo of a formula manufacturer, I felt like a fraud, too healthy to deserve the stuff because I wasn't really a new mother. I wasn't shuffling my feet across the floor, suffering with an episiotomy, or bent with an abdominal incision. My hair wasn't sticking up every which way. My face didn't have the wan, happy exhaustion of the post-partum woman who is proud of her accomplishment. But if they wanted to give me sample cans of extra-strength formula, a box of preemie-sized diapers, and the latest edition of a magazine for new mothers, I would take it.

The nurse taped a diaper into place across Sarah's belly and then slipped the gown over her head. The fabric had a pale white background that was dotted with pink chicks, and I'd noticed the softness when I'd folded and packed it into the bag. The fabric was almost not palpable to the fingertips. The nurse talked quietly to Sarah as she eased one delicate baby arm and then the other into sleeves still too long. Sarah needed a pre-preemie size. Grandma's pink booties completed the outfit but were soon tucked inside the gown cinched with a drawstring at the bottom. When the dress-up was complete, the nurse placed her hand behind Sarah's back and moved her into a sitting position in the isolette. Sarah peered out unhappily from under a hat that matched the gown and then decided that the best course was to close her eyes.

Unlike the excitement surrounding her arrival at the hospital, Sarah's departure was not dramatic. It was anticlimactic but not a disappointment. Just weird, that Sarah's discharge could be so unremarkable. How was it possible I could simply walk out of the hospital with this baby? The lack of fanfare made me feel as if I were doing something illegal and trying to make a getaway without being noticed, much like the time I had made the great escape from my room at Baystate. As I stood in front of the elevator doors with the nurse carrying Sarah per the hospital's rules, I was tempted to look back over my shoulder to see if anyone was following us, someone wanting to reclaim my baby.

We stepped out of the elevator and I broke ahead of the nurse's careful pace and jogged to the car. As I unlocked the door and slipped into the driver's seat, the thought occurred to me that although it had been a good idea to send Willie away for this weekend, it had been a mistake to let Jeff go.

Damn, Susan, you are a nutcase, I thought. Now that it was happening, I realized that Sarah's homecoming was not a moment I should be experiencing on my own. I felt a gap left by Jeff's absence. I wished he were the one sitting behind the steering wheel and I was standing on the sidewalk in the brilliant sunshine and waiting for him to drive up for me and Sarah.

Maybe you can get it together after today, I thought. Maybe you can believe in this baby, as Jeff always has, and stop being so anxious. Just maybe.

Looking over my shoulder, I backed the car out of its place. The last time, I thought. This is the last time I am sitting in this car in this parking lot without my baby in her car seat.

When I pulled up to the hospital entrance and stepped out of the car, I saw a woman I recognized. She worked for Health Choice, the HMO we belonged to, the one that was paying Sarah's considerable hospital bills. I searched for a name. Jackie. She was supporting an elderly woman on one arm, and both women looked up as I walked over to open the door on the passenger side where the car seat was strapped in and ready.

Jackie had been nothing like the stereotype of the impersonal insurance company employee. She had been as sympathetic as a therapist when I called her with questions about coverage for Sarah's hospitalization, and, more recently, about the equipment we would need at home. The nurse, still holding Sarah, stood poised to place her in the infant seat. As Jackie made her way slowly up the sidewalk, her eye landed first on Sarah. Her face softened in the inevitable response of many women when they see babies. Before I could speak, Jackie looked from the baby to me and back to the baby and then covered her mouth with her hand. Her eyes filled with tears, surprising both of us, and she was speechless, continuing to press her fingers to her mouth as she tried to compose herself. She finally breathed, "Oh . . . is this . . . ?" as she tilted her head sideways to get a straight-on view of the little bit of face showing from under the hat and above the blanket.

When she found her voice again, Jackie introduced her mother and attempted to tell an abridged version of Sarah's life story. As she talked, Jackie found a tissue and dabbed at her eyes.

Sarah did not rise to the occasion. In fact, she was looking a little crabby, a frown wrinkling her forehead and her eyes tightly shut against the sun and newness of the outdoors. It didn't matter. Jackie could see through Sarah's mood. I told Jackie when she went back to work on Monday morning, she should let Health Choice know that its money had been well spent.

After fastening Sarah into her infant seat, I thanked the nurse who had escorted us to the parking lot, then sat myself in the front seat of the car, and waved goodbye to the nurse, Jackie, and her mother. Once my seatbelt was firmly snapped across my lap—every step seemed to have exaggerated importance as if I were taking off in an airplane—I put the gearshift into drive and stepped on the gas. I turned the car right out of the hospital lot and left onto High Street. We headed for home.

So strange to have her in the car with me. So normal to drive past Agway and the dry cleaner with my baby in her seat. We were driving home on a Saturday morning as if it were nothing special, and I wondered how she could possibly be the little creature who had been born in January. I kept peeking sideways. Her eyes were still tightly closed, but I didn't believe she was really asleep. The discharge social worker who worked with NICU parents warned me that because the baby resented the assault of light and noise in the NICU, she would very quickly shut down to activity that she found excessive. When it reached a level too loud, too light, too much, she might not necessarily cry but would withdraw and just drop out of the scene by closing her eyes. That was what she was doing in the car. Beneath the silly cap, I could see scrunched eyelids and an otherwise unreadable face. I drove gingerly, feeling as if the moment were breakable.

When I turned off Route 2, Miss Weed, the golden retriever and sometimes guard dog, was positioned uncharacteristically in the center of the driveway as if she did not want to miss our arrival. I would have to run over her in order to get to the garage, so I stopped in the driveway. She came around to my car door with a wagging tail. I was glad to have someone to talk to.

"Look, Miss Weed! Look who's here!" I got out of the car and patted Miss Weed, and we went over to Sarah's side. Opening the door, I looked down at a baby who looked no different from any other newborn. I unhooked her seat belt, disengaged the entire package of baby and seat, eased it out of the car, and walked into the kitchen. I set the car seat on the counter.

The kitchen seemed dark until my eyes adjusted from the bright light outdoors. The house was unnaturally quiet without Willie and Jeff. I wasn't sure what to do next. The nurse had given Sarah a bottle just before I'd arrived at the hospital, so it wasn't yet time for a feeding. There was no movement under the pink quilt that covered her, and she kept her eyes closed.

"You're here, Sarah. You're home now." No response from the sleeping baby. The dog recognized that even though we were in the kitchen, there wasn't going to be any cooking in the foreseeable future. She moved to her favorite corner, turned around a few times, and lay down. I stood before Sarah, the four-month-old, now four-pound baby who lay serenely in her infant seat on my kitchen counter. I watched her breathe.

Seeing that the baby intended to be quiet in this new place, I took her out of the seat and settled her into the cradle Jeff's dad had built for Willie. It was a honey-colored maple, fashioned to gently rock a baby to sleep. Puz had been smart enough to know, however, that eventually a big brother like Willie could give a future sibling more than a quiet swing. As clever as he was creative, Puz had carved wooden keys at both ends of the cradle to lock it into place. I had felt sad and a little guilty that Puz had put so much effort into the cradle. Willie had slept in it for barely three months before his arms and legs grew too long for its dimensions. He would wake up with his head jammed in the corner and marks from the bars denting a pattern on his forehead.

Sarah, I figured, would be in the cradle for a while.

After she slept for a few hours, drank from a bottle, and had her diaper changed—routine activities that seemed anything but routine on that day—I picked her up and stepped outside to take a walk through the yard. She seemed weightless. Not even as heavy as a bag of sugar. The air was so mellow she didn't have to stay all bundled up, and I spread a blanket on the grass and lay her on it. I opened the string on the bottom of her gown to remove the booties so she could feel the afternoon air on her feet and legs. Miss Weed was all attention and walked the property with us. When I placed the baby on the blanket, Miss Weed circled a few times and then lay down in a good resting spot. I talked quietly to Sarah, and eventually the softness of the new sounds must have seemed safe. She opened her dark eyes for the first time since leaving the hospital.

Every moment of the day was a joy. I was sorry Jeff wasn't with us but also found comfort in the solitude. Hours passed, and I didn't turn on the radio or TV or any of the things that would connect me to the world. The phone didn't ring. I ate a light supper and cleaned up in just a few minutes. We settled in for the evening. The long May day took its time to wind down, and by the time the sun moved behind the trees, Sarah lay peacefully sleeping in her cradle. Her face was finally relaxed, and I knew she was really asleep and not just pulling the curtain on the outside world. I did not turn any lights on. I sat in a chair next to the cradle, rocked it quietly with one hand, and patted the dog's worried head with the other. I hummed a lullaby to both of them. As dark came over the room, the only light to be seen was the rhythmic flicker of green on the apnea monitor assuring me that for the first time in 131 days all was well.

ISOLATION

Sunday was a day for Sarah and me to get to know one another. I didn't have much of a sense of time that day. I didn't do much around the house. I was pretty well organized anyway. I had shopped for groceries on Friday evening, so we were stocked with food and supplies for Muz's visit. Sarah moved from wakefulness to her naps and was quietly present, never fussy. I offered her the breast at feeding times, but she didn't act interested, and I didn't want to stress her or make her unhappy while she was adjusting to her home. I squelched my niggling anxiety about whether or not she would ever nurse.

The quiet was lovely, but by the end of the day I'd had quite enough tranquility. Jeff, Willie, and Muz were due home late that evening, and I was ready to turn on the dancing music, ready for the three generations of Blomstedts to get home and spice the place up. I wanted Sarah to step into the picture of the family I had been visualizing for five months.

Dusk was falling over the smooth waters of the cove when the phone rang. It was Jeff. This was in the pre-cell phone era, so he was calling from a pay phone at a highway rest stop somewhere in New Jersey.

"Hi, Hon," he hollered. He sounded as if he was talking from the far end of a tin can. "I just wanted to call and warn you." A pause. "Willie has a temperature of 103."

Oh, no, I thought, but couldn't think of what to say for a moment. "Oh, no," I then said aloud.

"No rash or anything," he continued loudly. "He did vomit. But only once."

Oh, swell, I thought.

"Lucky I have Muz with me," he said to my silence.

"For sure," I answered. Then I said, "Poor guy," not knowing who to worry about first.

I was concerned about Willie, of course, but this development threw a wrench into the plans.

I had to ask Jeff, "What should we do with the baby? We can't expose her to a virus."

"I guess we'll just have to keep Willie away from her for now," he said.

"But how will we do that?" I asked. "If Willie knows the baby is here, he'll be all over her."

"I don't know how to do it," he answered, sounding a little belea-guered. "We'll have to figure something out. Anyway, the traffic has been pretty heavy. We won't be home until around midnight," he said and signed off.

Because we wanted to keep the baby close to us when she came home, I had asked Jeff to put her cradle in our bedroom, which was on the main floor of the house. To get to the bathroom, all traffic had to pass through our bedroom, defining it as a main thoroughfare. Willie traveled that route all day. The way the house was set up made it difficult to keep him away from his sister.

And how would I keep myself from getting sick? Since Willie had been born, I had managed to catch just about every cold he'd sniffled through. As compulsive and frequent as my hand washing might be, I had been unsuccessful at avoiding his illnesses.

There had to be a way to stay healthy. I wandered around the house, trying to think of how. There were two bedrooms upstairs. Willie slept in one, and the other we used as a guestroom. Muz would be staying there.

Then I had a thought.

Beyond the bedroom section of the house's second story was one of the quirkier features of our thirty-eight-year-old dwelling. It was a long, wide space that was essentially the house's attic. It was as big as a room, but the ceiling was so low that even I couldn't stand up straight in it, and I'm only five feet, four inches tall. It was kind of an intriguing space, its floor covered with a 1970s vintage orange, indoor-outdoor style carpeting. It even had an electrical outlet. It was the kind of place I could picture the kids playing in when they were older, holding meetings of secret societies or performing plays in a room made to scale for its occupants. It was a room where the miniature tables and chairs in Lynda's kitchen would be in the proper proportion, a late twentieth-century version of the attic where Jo, Meg, Beth, and Amy spent their winter afternoons in *Little Women*.

The room in the attic stretched above the entire space of the kitchen, dining area, and master bedroom, so, I concluded, it was plenty big enough for me and the baby to camp in for a few days. Muz could take care of Willie. He wouldn't even have to know I was at home, and when he recovered from his illness, we could have a reunion. I knew I couldn't protect Sarah from colds and common childhood sicknesses in-definitely, but she'd been home for less than forty-eight hours. It wasn't right to challenge her immune system by exposing her to Willie's illness so soon. Muz needed the guestroom, so that left the attic as my only choice. I would do what I could to keep myself and the baby isolated until Willie was no longer contagious. I didn't know if I was being clever or crazy, but until someone else had a better suggestion, the baby and I would be moving to the attic.

It had been a long time since I'd used a playpen for Willie, but I found it in a closet off the kitchen and lugged it up the stairs. I lined it with blankets and a flannel sheet and set up the apnea monitor on the floor next to the temporary bed. Around ten o'clock, I woke Sarah to feed and change her and then carried her up to her new bed. I unscrambled the two wires that dangled from underneath her gown, plugged them into the back of the monitor, and turned the machine on. She immediately resumed the sleep she had been enjoying before I'd disturbed her. I moved the Fisher Price intercom that was usually in Willie's room to where Sarah was now situated and looked around at my setup. I'd pulled a mattress out of the corner and placed it on the floor for myself, and there was an electrical outlet where I could plug in the apnea monitor and a lamp for reading. No scrubbing or sterile gowns were required for entry into our space. It wasn't luxurious but the ceiling was insulated, the floor was carpeted and clean, and I felt we were safe from marauding microorganisms. We were separated from the general travel patterns of our household, and that's what I wanted.

I walked down the stairs to await the return of the rest of my family. I turned on the intercom in the kitchen but heard only silence from upstairs where Sarah lay sleeping in my homemade isolation ward.

When the weary travelers finally arrived, it was close to midnight. Willie was asleep, and his eyes stayed closed when Jeff carried him up to his room. I hugged Muz as she walked in with hands full of diaper bag and whatnots. She returned a wan smile. I knew it must have been a rough trip. I carried her suitcase to her room. Then I walked across the hall to Willie's bedroom door and watched as Jeff got the little guy settled in his crib. Germs or no, I couldn't have Willie in the house and not at least see him. I knew from the flushed cheeks that his face and head were hot with fever. Jeff wakened Willie just enough to give him the liquid Tylenol I'd poured into a plastic measuring cup. Willie cried a little, a low, irritable whine that sounded as if he had a sore throat, but he didn't protest for long. He drank the medicine and lay back down. He was soon asleep.

I led Jeff and Muz down the hall to Sarah's special room. The last time Muz had seen Sarah was on Easter weekend when she and Puz had come for a holiday visit. She watched the sleeping baby and said in her southern drawl, "Oh, my goodness. Just look at that doll-baby." I walked downstairs with her and Jeff to catch up on events of the weekend and the hell-ride back. It had only gotten worse, both traffic and vomiting, after Jeff and I had talked on the phone. Neither of them was feeling particularly chatty at that late and weary hour, and we retired to our rooms. The happy tableau that I envisioned for their return faded into the background to wait for a better day.

On Monday, Muz took charge of Willie's care. He sounded as if he was feeling a little better, and his temperature was lower than the night before although it spiked again in the late afternoon. Muz said he didn't tug at his ears or show any sign of a rash or other symptoms, so she was just going to keep an eye on him and let me know if anything worrisome cropped up.

On Monday evening, I realized after Willie and his germs went to bed, there was no reason for Sarah and me to stay upstairs. When I could hear some regularity to the tune whistling through Willie's stuffy nose, I tiptoed past his room and down the stairs with Sarah in my arms. We visited with Muz and Jeff, who sat together in the living room. The TV was on, but neither was watching it. Muz worked on a pile of laundry. We talked as we folded and stacked. Jeff read the newspaper. I'd figured out that, with Willie all the way upstairs, Sarah could sleep in her cradle in the master bedroom without being threatened and I could sleep in my own bed. Our isolation was not complete with this plan, but it seemed effective enough as long as we stayed away from Willie's germs.

By Tuesday Willie's illness had blossomed into a full-blown head cold, but the fever was gone. Through their ceiling—my floor—I could hear Muz as she talked her grandson through the process of making a batch of chocolate chip cookies. Muz was being a good sport, trying to make sense of Willie's language. Her experience with her own five children came in handy that day. In addition to paying attention to Willie, she washed more clothes, started dinner preparations, and sneaked up the stairs with an afternoon cup of tea and more laundry for me to fold.

By the time Wednesday morning dawned, I'd had enough of the attic. I was having a hard time maintaining the frantic sense of urgency about Sarah's health and Willie's contagion I'd felt on Sunday evening. Who knew how long Willie could have a cold? The average cold lasts ten to fourteen days. Muz would be with us for only a week. After some hours of ruminating over the pros and cons of the next course of action, I carried Sarah downstairs, joined the family, and resolved that I would do what I could to keep Willie from breathing on his sister or me.

141

In the end I suffered a defeat in my battle with the germs. On Thursday evening I noticed that Sarah's nose seemed a bit stuffy. On Friday, she was congested enough to give her trouble with feeding. The roses had disappeared from her cheeks, and she seemed tired, especially when she tried to eat. She couldn't suck and breathe at the same time. I knew her condition was deteriorating when she became so frustrated with feeding that she cried. It was the first time she'd cried since coming home, and when I thought about it, I realized it was the first time I'd ever heard her cry. I suppose there were times she could have cried when she was in the hospital, but she'd had few painful procedures after being extubated so there wasn't much reason for her to cry. She'd been calm and mellow from her first moments at home.

On Saturday morning, when the apnea monitor alarmed and then alarmed a second time, I knew the illness was affecting her breathing enough to exhaust her. Even though I suctioned out her tiny nostrils with the pink rubber bulb provided by the hospital, it wasn't enough. She couldn't drink much from a bottle with such a stuffy nose. I took her temperature and found she had developed a low-grade fever. I began to worry about the illness in general and about dehydration in particular.

Jeff and Willie were driving Muz to the train station that morning, so I was home alone with Sarah. I gave up trying to manage her illness on my own and called the pediatrics office. Unfortunately, Hugh was off for the weekend. I fretted about having to take Sarah to one of his partners. Will I have to explain her entire history? Will he understand her fragility and the urgency of her situation?

Fifteen minutes after I made the phone call asking for an appointment, we were in an exam room. It didn't take long for me to figure out that Hugh's partner was well versed on Sarah's history. Of course, partners would talk to one another about a case like Sarah's. I should have known that. I also should have had more confidence in the level of mindfulness the doctor would bring to his exam of a sick baby, mine or anyone's. Each baby requires the same attention from the pediatrician, and every one is special.

Hugh's partner was very thorough in his exam, his eyes all over the baby as he asked me questions, his large hands brown against her skin as he gently positioned her on the exam table. He placed the diaphragm of his stethoscope to her chest, her back, her chest again while he cocked his head and listened intently. When he finished, he didn't order blood work or hand me a prescription.

He straightened up and said, "I think it would be best if we put her in the hospital."

Damn, I thought. Though I knew the doctor was being thorough and appropriately conservative, that wasn't the answer I wanted.

Trying not to think about what was happening, I quickly dressed Sarah, scooped her into my arms, slung the diaper bag over my shoulder, and headed back out to the parking lot. I packed us into the car and drove the three miles from the doctor's office to the hospital. Jeff and Willie wouldn't be back from the train station yet, so I couldn't even call home, but Jeff probably wouldn't be surprised by the news.

The nurses on the pediatrics floor at Franklin Medical Center were waiting for their new admission, oxygen tent set up and already filled with steam by the time we arrived. They weren't happy Sarah was sick, of course, but they did not hide their delight about having her as their charge. One nurse took Sarah from me, and I could hear cooing and sweet-talk going on as their shadows moved inside the steamy tent. Over the course of the day, the nurses performed their rituals. They drew blood with some difficulty, and Sarah cried at that. They gave her nebulizer treatments. She coughed. She slept. She coughed some more. She took a little electrolyte solution from a bottle. She wheezed, coughed, and looked unhappy.

It took a week of living in an oxygen tent to bring her back, a week of nurses hovering, suctioning, and giving breathing treatments and medicines. I drove back and forth, and Willie went back to Lynda's on his old schedule. Once Muz was back in Pennsylvania and Sarah back in the hospital, it seemed that nothing had changed in our lives as if the few days when Sarah was home had been just a wish.

It took a week, and then she came home once again. I took deep, calming breaths. Once again my family started what I hoped would be a life at home with Sarah.

BOTTLE VS. BREAST: ROUND TWO

On the Saturday after Sarah returned home from the hospital the second time without a fever but still coughing a little, I decided, this is it: now or never. The time had come when I would seriously begin the breast-feeding lessons. All of the conditions were in place, and I had no other "if onlys" to use as excuses.

Though I kept tucking the worry away, I was becoming increasingly anxious about this moment because I saw it as a last chance to hold onto the one possible physical connection I could have with Sarah. I had hoped when she left Baystate and came to the hospital near home we could begin to have some breast-feeding time together. When Sarah was in the nursery at Franklin Medical Center, a nurse who specialized in breast-feeding problems helped me with ideas, equipment, positioning, quiet rooms, and whatever she could think of to set the scene and make things work. Sarah wasn't interested. When she turned her head away from me, I continued to rationalize: this will be better when she comes home. We will be relaxed and calm. We will have privacy in our quiet house without strangers walking in and out of the room. Then I will hold her close and she will turn to me and we will make up for all the time that we've missed. I don't know where Willie was in that serene, private picture.

I knew Sarah would be my last child. If the doctors couldn't tell me why I'd developed an infection and this baby was born prematurely, I could not put another baby through a beginning like Sarah's. That fact made nursing all the more important to me. I wanted her to have the best nourishment possible, this baby who thus far had almost no experiences natural for a baby in the first year of her life. I wanted her to be healthy. I wanted her to have the antibodies from breast milk. Mostly, I wanted to sit on the sofa and snuggle with her for her feedings each day. Bottle-feeding a baby didn't fulfill that need for me.

I set my plan into motion. Since it was the weekend, Jeff was home to help care for Willie. There would be no bottles on this day, I decided. I would offer only the breast for each feeding. When she got hungry enough, I knew she would nurse. Her instinct was to survive. I had tried nursing her during her first week home from the hospital when we were in the attic, but she refused and I hadn't pushed her with real conviction. I didn't want to admit in that first week at home that we might be beyond the point of no return.

Now it was time to get serious. I mentally clenched my teeth and prepared for what I wanted to be the joy of nursing my baby.

That afternoon, when she fussed a bit with a sound that I interpreted as hunger, I carried Sarah into the living room where we settled comfortably on the sofa. Twenty minutes earlier I had wrestled in the kitchen with a new contraption that would supposedly help Sarah get used to nursing. Because sucking from the breast requires so much more energy than sucking from a bottle—especially the preemie bottle Sarah was used to, one with a soft nipple that had lots of tiny slits in its tip—a nurse at the hospital had introduced me to a setup that would reward Sarah with an easy flow of milk from the bottle as she learned to suck from the breast.

First, I filled a pint-sized plastic bottle with two ounces of warmed breast milk. Bags of it, begging to be used, still tumbled out of my freezer. I hung the bottle on an IV pole I borrowed from the hospital. I opened the clamp. The flexible tubing that extended from the bottle filled with milk. When milk began dripping from the end of the tubing, I clamped it off and wheeled the IV pole with the bottle dangling over my head into the living room.

When Sarah and I sat down on the sofa together, I laid her flat for a minute so I could manipulate the end of the tubing to make it protrude along the contour of my nipple. I then taped it to my breast so it would stay in place. If all went well, Sarah would get tubing and nipple simultaneously. Over time I should be able to decrease the flow of milk by adjusting the clamp, and she would gradually tug with enough strength to be fed from the breast alone.

The morning had started warm for June, and the air only got hotter and stickier in the afternoon. The house was quiet. Jeff had taken Willie outside to work on a project, which I appreciated, but I had no extra hands to help me. I positioned Sarah in the curve of my right arm while with my left hand I struggled to organize tube, nipple, and baby mouth. Sarah sniffed around at my right breast for a bit and then turned away. I tried again to get her into position, face turned, mouth to breast, where milk dribbled out of the tubing. Clearly making a choice, she flipped her head back. I felt my skin break into a sweat as if the temperature in the room had just risen another ten degrees. I was perspiring, not just under my arms, but also on my scalp, my forehead, my neck, and between my breasts.

I put Sarah down on the cushion again, removed the tape from my right breast, and moved everything over to the left. Some babies have preferences and will nurse on one side and not the other. I tucked her into position once more.

"Come on, Sarah," I purred, believing Sarah would hear the soothing and not recognize the grim determination. "Come on, Sweetie. This is good." She wiggled, not cooperatively. Milk continued to dribble from the tubing and formed rivulets that leaked onto my shorts. When I moved or adjusted my position, droplets of milk flew from the tubing and then stood in white beads on the amber sofa fabric. My breast hung out in the open. Without a free hand, I turned my head to wipe my sweaty face on the shoulder of my shirt.

"This is good, Sweetie Pie, just try. You'll be surprised. Come on, try it."

But she would not. She arched her back and turned her head, her face bright red and wet with her own perspiration. Finally, after I re-positioned her again and lined her mouth up with the equipment, she opened her mouth and screamed in frustration. I had never heard her cry like that.

I allowed my body to fall back on the sofa and felt my face crumple. Some goals in life respond to grim determination, but breast-feeding a baby is probably not one. I sat for a while, crying. Then I wiped my nose on the other sleeve of my tee shirt. Tears mixed with the droplets of sweat I could feel on my face.

I pulled my shirt down. The battle was over, and it felt to me as if we were both losers.

I could hear the back door slam as the guys came inside. Jeff, wondering whether or not he had heard his cue, poked his head into the living room.

"Here. You take her," I said, lifting her five-and-a-half pounds, offering her up. Jeff walked up to me and reached out for the crying baby. Knowing there was not a thing he could say that would be right, he looked at me. I broke the silence and spoke the words of my surrender, "I'll go and fix a bottle."

ONE MORNING IN JUNE

Willie's crib was in his room on the second floor, and over the intercom in my bedroom I could hear him murmuring quietly to himself in the softening light of the morning. After some moments of silence, he hollered. "Ma!"

Ten seconds of silence. Then, "Mom?"

Another quiet moment. Then, "Mom!"

Five forty-five. From under one eyelid I could see the red numbers on the clock radio. Jeff did not hear the intercom on that June morning. Or maybe he did not respond because his name was not "Mom!" In either case, he remained on his left side, his back to me, his breathing quiet and regular. I pushed back the covers, swung my legs over the side of the bed, and sat there for a moment.

"Mom!"

In the far corner of our bedroom, all I could see of the contents of the cradle were a yellow gingham bumper and an edge of the pink flannel quilt my sister Lorie had made for Sarah back in February. Lorie had embroidered each of the quilt's two-inch squares with a different motif: a bow and a heart, a flower and a butterfly, a squash racquet and a building block labeled with the letters SKB. To give Sarah some relief from the relentless fluorescence of the NICU, the nurses used the quilt to cover the top of the isolette at night. In her cradle at home, Sarah lay quietly under the undisturbed surface of the quilt. She hadn't cried in the night. She hadn't wakened to be fed. She slept in complete peace. She was making up, I believed, for the first 130 nights of her life.

The apnea monitor green light flashed each time she took a breath. "Mom!"

No time for lingering sentimentality. The voice was persistent.

I turned the intercom speaker off and shuffled up the stairs to retrieve the source of the hollering. Waiting for him to notice me, I peeked my head around the door of Willie's bedroom. Though the light was still subdued, I could clearly see him as he stood gripping the rail of his crib with both hands, knuckles white, measuring the time interval until he should produce his next shout. Since he didn't know many words, timing and volume were key. He jumped up and down when he saw me.

"Good morning, Little Guy." He smiled and bounced a few more times for good measure.

Groaning noisily, I lifted him over the rail. He anchored himself on me by wrapping his long legs around my waist and an arm around my neck. His diaper weighs as much as he does, I thought. Two kids in diapers. That had never been in the grand plan. But here I was, a thirty-two-year-old mother walking down the stairs, carrying a toddler in giant Pampers and then peeking in the cradle at the infant who still did not fit into a preemie-sized diaper.

I know parents who actually get up with their children at five thirty in the morning. They fill the coffee pot, break out the cereal boxes, and start the day when their kids wake up. Jeff and I were attempting to teach Willie that the day did not start at such an ungodly hour. "This is a quiet time," we told him each day at five thirty.

After a diaper change, Willie joined the still-sleeping Jeff in our bed. I did give in somewhat to Willie's wakefulness. I gathered a few picture books, some kind of vehicle with four wheels, and a puzzle. Then I reassumed the horizontal. When Jeff rolled over after a half hour of Willie's play, I saw a cow shape stuck to his shoulder. Delighted to have rediscovered it, Willie peeled the piece off his daddy's skin.

Jeff eventually gave up the pretense of sleep and responded to the poking and nose-pulling. Willie squealed through a bout of tickling and wrestling that resulted in a general disruption of sheets and blankets. When the giggling subsided, Jeff remembered who he needed to be on that day and, in his face and his posture, assumed the responsibilities of the next thirteen hours. He headed for the shower, and in twenty minutes he was dressed and out the door.

I heard a few squeaks coming from the cradle and told Willie it was time for his sister to start the day, too. That was a bath morning. Splashing in the tub always made Willie happy. I decided I might as well bathe Sarah, too, since I had to weigh her. When Sarah was discharged from the hospital, the visiting nurse loaned us a scale to keep track of Sarah's weight until she showed a consistent, positive trend. Sarah weighed four pounds when she came home from Franklin Medical Center, and although she had lost some ground when she spent a week in the hospital at the end of May, she had since gained steadily.

Willie stepped into the bath and moved immediately onto his belly in order to get his lips to the water for bubble blowing. Sarah lay on the changing table with a plastic strap fastened across her belly. She stared at the Mother Goose figures hanging on the wall while I ran warm water into the plastic tub on the bathroom counter next to the sink. I could bathe Sarah and watch Willie at the same time.

When Sarah was undressed, there was not much to her, but she looked complete. Miniature but softly rounded and well-nourished. I lifted her from the changing table and set her in the yellow tub. Her belly moved in and out with the shock of the water, and she waved her arms and legs as if trying to remember if this was something she liked. Apparently deciding that the bath was okay after all, she settled in and stopped waving.

I used a washcloth to trickle warm water over her chest and arms. It was interesting to me that when she moved her arms and legs, it wasn't with the jerky, spasmodic motion of a newborn. Her nervous system was more sophisticated than that, and her movements showed some maturity. Scars from IVs were sprinkled over her wrists, the insides of her elbows, and the backs of her hands like a dot-to-dot leading to no recognizable picture. When I moved the washcloth around her scalp, I could see the area behind her ear still looked rough and irregular as if it had been burned. The rough spot was where the central IV line had poked out from under her skin for over two months.

I dipped the cloth in the warm water and rubbed her legs, and she wriggled with the newness of sensations that surrounded her. I wet her feet, rubbed her heels, and remembered. When Sarah was in the NICU, the sight of her heels made me feel sick. With a constellation of comma-sized wounds in various stages of healing, her heels had been raw from repeated blood drawing. On that morning in June, I massaged her scarred heels in the warm water and thought how the hard, bumpy surfaces were so unlike what a baby's should be. She curled her toes.

While I lingered over Sarah, Willie sloshed around in the tub. Knowing his contentment would run itself out as soon as the water cooled, I lifted Sarah from her bath and wrapped her in a white towel with a duck embroidered on one corner. That towel had wrapped around Willie for only a few weeks before his arms and legs were sticking out in all directions and we had to move on to something bigger. There was no threat of Sarah outgrowing the ducky towel anytime soon. Holding her in one arm, I leaned over the edge of the tub to pull the plug on Willie's bath. The water temperature had dropped, and he did not resist taking my hand to get out.

Dripping on the bath mat, he shivered loudly, forcing his teeth into a chatter. Still holding Sarah, I grabbed a big towel from the shelf and wrapped Willie up, too. I rubbed him with my free hand until he was dry. Now the two of them had shiny noses and stand-up wet hair. His was fair and stood in punky spikes; hers was fine and soft, toweled into swirls ending in fine, dark tips.

Though Willie's bedroom was upstairs, I kept his clothes on shelves in the downstairs bathroom. I rifled through the shelves with one hand and held Sarah with the other. When Willie was finally dressed in shorts and a striped shirt, he toddled into the bedroom in search of the morning's next adventure. Miss Weed, poor thing, lay in a corner and apparently appeared to Willie to be the perfect friend. He turned himself around and sat down, quite deliberately and carefully, on top of her.

I turned back to the bathroom. Placing a dry washcloth on the baby scale, I balanced it to zero. Then I carefully placed Sarah on her tummy on the tray. She did not protest as she had when David weighed her in the NICU but lay quietly, eyes tolerant with her head turned towards me. What could be going on behind such serious eyes? The needle on the scale bobbed up and down, settled, then stopped. I bent down and turned my head sideways to be sure I saw it right. The needle pointed clearly to the number six. Six pounds in June, five months after she was born. A personal best. From a starting weight the equivalent of six sticks of butter, she could now share the seesaw with an entire bag of sugar and even a little more.

LOVE IS A VERY LIGHT THING

From January through April, I had written occasional newsletters to our cross-country friends to update them on Sarah's status. I sent the last note in the mail on the day Sarah moved from Baystate to the hospital in Greenfield. After that letter, there were no more newsletters from Gill. We'd been too busy getting organized, traveling back and forth from the hospital, and then just figuring out how to live with two kids. As the June days passed, we no longer had a reason to delay sending the official announcement of Sarah's birth. It looked as if she was with us for the long haul, and it was about time we let everyone know.

Jeff and I had been prompt about getting Willie's birth announcement in the mail. We had only three weeks from the day he was born to the day the moving van was coming to move us back east. We needed to complete the announcement before we left Wenatchee because we knew we faced weeks of unpacking when we reached Massachusetts.

Willie and I came home from the hospital on a Sunday afternoon, and at seven o'clock Monday morning, Jeff was setting up the scene for the photo shoot. The July morning held the threat of another thermometer-breaking day, but at that early hour the air was still comfortable enough. Everything seemed to have a golden glow in those first hours I spent at home with my new baby. I thought this would be a sweet moment with Jeff snapping a few pictures of the new baby to place in cards to friends. It soon became apparent, however, that Jeff's standards for the project were different from mine.

With a furrowed brow, he stared at our bed. He was already dressed in shirt and tie for work, which made him seem all the more serious. I helped him pull up the sheets and smooth the bedspread, and he placed a blue blanket on top of that. Then he set out on a mission. I heard kitchen drawers open and slam shut. He scuttled down the basement stair. There was silence, and I heard him take the steps two at a time. Out to the garage and back in. The car door opened and closed. Every now and then he returned to the bedroom and added something to the heap on the bed. He reminded me of the father in *Cheaper by the Dozen* as he approached what should have been the joyful task of taking a family portrait and went at it like an army general.

When Jeff was satisfied with his collection, he began to arrange the things he'd gathered in some formation on the bed. I asked if I could help, but no. He had a vision.

After making a preliminary layout of the items, Jeff lifted the sleeping baby out of his cradle and set him down in the center of the blue blanket. He smoothed the fabric under the miraculously sleeping Willie. Then he started moving again, carefully rearranging the things he hoped would fill his son's life. For music he had a ukulele and a harmonica in their artistically correct places. A hammer indicated the child would be skilled with his hands. Sports were well represented by a golf ball and putter, fishing rod and reel, a horseshoe, squash racket, and a ski pole. For a pillow, Jeff gently lifted Willie's head and allowed it to settle back into the sweet spot of a baseball glove. The baby looked as if he'd spent his nine months in utero dreaming about resting his head in just such a place.

To complete the scene and to acknowledge the hoped-for intellectual as well as athletic prowess of this boy, Jeff placed a pair of wire-rimmed eyeglasses, a calculator, and three books in the upper left-hand corner of the photo. The title of the book on top is clearly visible, even in the photograph. *Great Expectations*.

Willie maintained the deep sleep of a just-fed newborn during the entire setup. In the photograph that we reprinted, his eyes are closed. Even so, he is wearing one of the half grins of infancy that makes him look as if he had a good joke he might share when the whole thing was over.

One week later the announcement was ready to go in the mail. The script that accompanied the photograph was printed in Jeff's calligraphic hand:

Great Expectations
from the
LITTLE DICKENS
William Joseph Blomstedt
12 July 1984   8# 4oz   22 in

Willie was official.

Having made such a production out of Willie's announcement, we felt obligated to announce Sarah's birth properly. Jeff's approach to the photo shoot was eerily similar to what I had observed on the morning when he'd done Willie's. I don't know why I expected it to be any different. Once we worked out the concept together, I stepped back. This announcement was supposed to be happy and lighthearted, but Jeff's face once again assumed a frown of concentration as he set off through the garage and house and rummaged around for the look he wanted to create. My job was to dress the baby and bring her to the designated spot and then to keep track of Willie. Jeff would do the rest, and that was okay with me.

He placed her on a blanket of pale pink on the lawn in the backyard. She wore a white cotton gown with a little pastel print pattern sprinkled over the fabric. I tied the ribbons of the matching bonnet underneath a chin that had actually developed a few fleshy folds. I wasn't sure I liked the bonnet, and we experimented with a number of hats until Sarah became what I could almost call cross, but who could blame her? It was a warm day, and this wasn't her idea of fun.

She was not smiling in the picture that made the final cut. Still in recovery mode, Sarah didn't do much smiling in her first weeks at home. Unlike the softly curling fingers of Willie's hands in his announcement picture, Sarah had a clenched left fist. The fingers of her right hand curled around the de-thorned stem of a red rose. I had clipped it that day from a bush in my garden that had produced a few blooms in spite of my neglect.

Sarah's announcement photo turned out to be less complex than Willie's. There were fewer props: only a blanket, a rose, and a baby dressed in an outfit with hat. We took eight or ten pictures, but we didn't need that many. Occasionally she blinked but was content to just be where she had been placed. She lay there, a quiet baby on a blanket on the grass in the yard under the shade of a maple tree.

One evening the following week, Jeff finished the dishwashing and then stood quietly thinking for a few minutes. He went to his desk, located his favorite fountain pen, and sat down at the kitchen counter. Adjusting the nib he'd chosen, he dabbed blue ink on a tissue that lay next to his elbow and made a Rorschach creation of blue splotches. Assuming his best penmanship posture, Jeff bent his head in concentration and touched his pen to the tissue one last time.

What he wrote first was one verse of a song, "Love is a Very Light Thing," from the Broadway musical *Fanny*. The lyrics fit Sarah as if they'd been written for her. "Love is a very light thing. Light as a song in the air. How do you start to fill up a heart? How many ounces there?" I remembered the time my dad had played the role of the Greek widower, Panisse, in a church production of *Fanny*. Panisse marries a young woman and is finally the proud bearer of a long-awaited son. In a scene when Panisse and his friend Cesar marvel over the boy, Cesar sings:

When the baby was born he weighed eight pounds,
Now he weighs twenty-three.
Where did they come from, those extra pounds?
What could they be?
Sixteen pounds of love, they are.
Sixteen solid pounds.
Sixteen pounds of caring and sharing and love.

After Sarah came home from the hospital, Cesar's words percolated in my mind. Where did the pounds come from? What could they be? How had she gained them? How had she survived against so many odds?

I answered my own questions. The pounds came from the months when the phone rang, when gifts arrived, when old friends brought frozen casseroles and Tupperware containers filled with soup all the way from New Haven, when I found offers for babysitting in the mailbox. Though I had felt lonely and bereft in the months after Sarah's birth, there was more support than I'd recognized at the time. Many people had been thinking about Sarah, pulling for her, praying for her, and sending strength to her, to Jeff, to me. When people had asked, "What can I do?" they meant it, but I hadn't known what to ask for. Even so, the caring, sharing, and love of friends and family had channeled through the hands of the nurses and doctors who had touched Sarah every day, and she survived because of all of them.

Jeff printed more of the song's words next to the place on the pink page where there would be a round photo of the little baby holding the rose:

Love is a very light thing.
Love is so fragile and frail.
You cannot hold it here in your hands
Or weigh it on a scale.
Dragonfly wings, that's all it is
Whispering by with no sound.
Oh, it takes a lot of love to make a pound.

On the inside of the card he printed:

Sarah Katherine Blomstedt
Debut: January 12, 1986
1 lb 9 oz 12 in
Release from protective custody:
May 17, 1986: 4 lb 1 oz
Now: 8 lb chubby
Latest quote: "I'll never be skinny again."

With that, Sarah was official.

SUMMERTIME, WHEN THE LIVING IS EASY

We settled into a life remarkable only for its normalcy. On a typical June morning, Jeff rose early and kissed the three of us goodbye, and I did what moms with two little kids do. First I changed diapers, one that held a quart and the other that held maybe a half cup. Then I fed Sarah while Willie sat in his high chair and worked over a breakfast of dry Cheerios. I dressed him in shorts and a tee shirt and her in a preemie-sized pastel outfit. I picked up toys that seemed to multiply when my back was turned. The three of us played on an old bedspread under the branches of the tall oaks and maples that shade our yard. On some days, we took short car trips to do errands, and we occasionally took long car trips to Cape Cod to see my parents at their summer place. We visited with my sister Lorie and her son Stephen who was a month younger than Willie. Sarah still needed medicines, and I took her to a weekly appointment with our pediatrician. The news was always good, and she seemed to be thriving. She sat in her infant seat on the kitchen counter and kept me company while I vacuumed the floor or washed the dishes or cooked with Willie, who stood on a kitchen chair and worked as sous chef. All seemed right with the world.

When Willie was a baby, the day's schedule revolved around his routine. I was surprised to learn that, even with Sarah in the picture, Willie continued to control the day. He was the one who had a schedule—a few mornings with Lynda each week, swim-and-gym class at the YMCA, visits to friends. Sarah's routine never became as regimented as Willie's had been. She slept in the car, drank from her bottle wherever we happened to be at feeding time, and accompanied me to the grocery store in the evening while I left Jeff to put Willie to bed. Before having children, I wondered about women with babies who unhurriedly squeezed the vegetables in the produce department of the grocery store at eight or nine o'clock in the evening. What kind of mother would take a baby out at such a time? Two kids later I knew: the kind of mother who had a baby and a toddler and wanted to hand the bedtime duties to Dad for an evening. As long as Sarah remained pleasantly portable, I packed her up and carried her wherever, whenever.

Willie's second birthday was approaching. July 12 was exactly six months from the day Sarah was born, and comparing their two birthdays was unavoidable. Sarah's would forever be associated with snow, winter parkas, and never-ending worry. Willie was born in the expansiveness of July with daylilies in the garden and sandals on our feet.

Willie was not such a terrible two, but he launched a few trial balloons every day as he looked over his shoulder to assure himself I was watching. While I was occupied with him, Sarah sat quietly in her seat or lay on the rag quilt my grandmother had pieced together years before she had ever thought there might be great-grandchildren in her life. The primary colors of the fabric tumbled over the living room floor, and Sarah never seemed bored as her bright eyes focused, day after day, on the diamond-shaped colors.

June was the month we left Sarah with her first out-of-hospital baby sitter. My youngest sister, Elaine, was to be married in June. She said all Jeff and I had to do was show up for the late afternoon ceremony since she knew we were not capable of more than that. I could hardly miss my sister's wedding, but what would I do with the baby? She was barely over six pounds, had been home from the hospital for only a few weeks, still needed medicines mixed into her formula every few hours, and was attached to the apnea monitor.

We would take her to the wedding, I decided. Elaine would have to understand. I wanted to be there, I wanted Jeff to be with me, and the baby's safety was the most important issue. We would sit in the back of the church if we had to. Sarah never made much noise anyway, I rationalized.

Then, two weeks before the wedding, the vision of a face floated across my consciousness like Mary Poppins under her umbrella. It was Deedy, a former NICU nurse and my telephone friend while Sarah was in the hospital. She and her family lived about ten miles away from where the wedding reception would be. I called to see if she would consider babysitting for Sarah on the night of Elaine's wedding. Deedy's three kids were all under the age of five, so this was a lot to ask. But I heard no hesitation at the end of the line.

"I'd love to do it," she said, "but there is one problem."

"Okay," I said. I thought she might have company or a scheduling conflict we would have to work around.

"I can't promise I'll give her back to you at the end of the evening."

Not wanting to overwhelm our friends and their brood, I arranged for Willie to stay with a sitter at home. We arrived at Patrick and Deedy's house an hour before the wedding was to begin. I felt like a nurse giving them report at the beginning of their shift.

"Here is her formula. I have two feedings ready in bottles. Here are her vitamins and the aminophylline she needs in her formula. She'll probably stay awake until around eight. Then you should be able to put her down. She doesn't usually cry." On and on. When I started to show Deedy the apnea monitor, I realized I had gone too far. She was well aware of how an apnea monitor worked. I shut my mouth, thanked her and Patrick profusely, and let Jeff drag me out the door. Deedy was a neonatal nurse, and her husband Patrick was an internist. The only way to find more competent babysitters would have been to put Sarah in the hospital for the evening.

In spite of knowing Sarah was in the best of hands and truly not worrying about her, I felt oddly removed from Elaine and Tim's wedding. I think Jeff did as well. We weren't quite ready to rejoin the world, not sure of our footing when it came to celebrating the good things in life. After the wedding ceremony and dinner, when people began to circulate from table to table and then worked their way towards the dance floor, I looked at Jeff, who looked as if he'd rather be anywhere but on the dance floor.

"Do you want to take a walk?" I asked him. He looked grateful for the invitation.

We slipped out of the room and stepped into the warmth of the June night. He took my hand and we walked, moving away from the cacophony of band, talk, and laughter. After a while, he started to talk about his dad. Puz was experiencing some worrisome physical symptoms.

Jeff's father had retired from his law career the year before Sarah was born. Since then he had spent his days keeping the lawns mowed and the house repaired. Then he rewarded himself with a round of golf. In March, while we were worrying about Sarah and oblivious to almost everything else, Puz noticed some fatigue and other vague symptoms. Until then, he'd had nothing more than an occasional cold or headache mar his good health. The thought of his being threatened with a serious illness seemed as impossible as if one of the carvings on Mount Rushmore had started to crumble. We exchanged phone calls with Muz through the spring, but she'd been sparing with the details and her worries, sympathetic to our tenuous hold on stability as Sarah made plodding progress. Puz went through some diagnostic testing in June. As life in Gill began to move into a warm current and my family entered into the festivities of Elaine's wedding day, the diagnosis from Puz's lymph node biopsy was still unclear. Maybe lymphoma, but the cells were not typical. The surgeon would have to sample another node and see if he could get a definite answer.

Jeff became quiet again, and I noticed that a familiar feeling, worry, had joined us on our stroll through the old New England village. Not knowing what to say next, we moved farther away from the strains of music that played on into the night of my sister's wedding.

On the weekend of July 4, we loaded up the red station wagon with the two kids and Miss Weed and set off on the seven-hour ride to the Blomstedt family home in Chadds Ford. I felt conflicted. Along with relief and the joy of being on a family trip with the family I had visualized for so many months, I also felt a profound fear about Puz's health.

We made the harrowing trip down the New Jersey Turnpike a few times each year, and I was always grateful when we made the final turn into the drive that led to the Blomstedt home. Jeff's parents lived on five acres, a wooded property surrounded by the bucolic, rolling countryside often painted by Andrew Wyeth. The first sight through the trees was the weathered old barn. That was where we would most likely find Puz, the place where he spent many hours dismantling and repairing a crotchety tractor that was probably as old as he. Beyond the barn a tall, narrow stone house rose out of the grassy hillside. Jeff parked the car. When I opened the door, the heat and humidity hit me like a baseball bat. Though New England summers have occasional stretches of days when the temperatures reach a hundred degrees and the muggy air leaves us sodden, the heat and humidity of eastern Pennsylvania is its own breed of weather. Ugh, was my only coherent thought. We found Muz in the blessedly air-conditioned kitchen where she distributed a month's worth of hugs and kisses. Then she led us up to a room on the second floor where all four of us could stay. It had wide pine boards that squeaked under our feet and a view of the pond from the dormer windows. After depositing the suitcases, Jeff took Sarah and left to find his dad in the barn. Muz took Willie back down to the kitchen for some lemonade and cookies, and I stayed in the guest room and organized our belongings.

Dinner was festive that evening as we were joined by Jeff's sisters, Martha and Phyllis, his brothers, Steve and Ed, and Ed's wife, Mae. Will adored his cousins, Eric and little Jeffrey, and the boys spent all but dinner time romping on the floor like three happy puppies.

No one could create a summer dinner like Muz. She was a native Floridian, and her southern roots were most apparent on steamy days when the menu reflected the foods she'd enjoyed as a girl. Puz seemed reassuringly like himself, if a little tired-looking. The family sipped cool drinks on the screened back porch, and everyone left the table satisfied. As the July sun mercifully descended behind the trees, a chorus of frogs started an evening performance at the pond's edge. Every now and again I could see the calm water ripple with a hint of the life that moved beneath its surface.

After breakfast on Saturday morning, I went back up to our room to dress Sarah. Willie was outside with Muz. Knowing he was in good hands, I walked back to where Sarah lay in the crib. Perhaps because I was away from home and could look at the morning routine in a different light, I noticed that in the two weeks since Sarah had turned six pounds, changes in her body seemed to be on fast-forward as if she were making up for lost time. I realized that the word "chubby," one I never thought would be in the same sentence as her name, could now be used to describe this baby. Her face was quite round, cheeks full, and she even had a double chin. I moved her to my bed and changed her diaper in a room that was already quite warm at eight in the morning. Beads of perspiration stood out on her forehead and glistened in the folds of her skin. Jeff emerged from a steamy bathroom shower with a towel wrapped around his waist and walked toward the dresser where he'd organized his clothes. He paused behind me and looked critically over my shoulder at Sarah.

"She sweats like a fat girl," he pronounced.

"That is an ungenerous, ungentlemanly, and even unfatherly thing for you to say," I said, taking the insult personally for Sarah.

Jeff grinned at my protestations and went off to dress. I felt a little miffed at him, but I had to admit that she did look . . . well . . . fat, and there was something about it, a puffiness, maybe, that bothered me. I shook off the feeling. I pressed the edges of a cloth diaper into the sweaty folds of Sarah's skin, told her she was beautiful just the way she was, and dressed her in a sunsuit for the hot day.

That day we learned from Muz that even after the second biopsy, the diagnosis for Jeff's dad remained unclear. Jeff, son and physician, picked up the phone. He called a friend in the pathology department at Yale whom he'd known from his training days, and the friend agreed to look at the slides. The pathologist said he would be in his office until three o'clock on Monday, so we needed to get there before then.

Since we had planned to leave on Monday, I didn't have a complaint about the timing, but I was a little annoyed with the plan. Driving the slides to Yale would have been a noble move if Jeff were on his own.

But tagging along were a toddler, a baby on an apnea monitor, a wife, a dog, and a station wagon weighed down with boxes, suitcases, and baby equipment. As if that weren't enough, we were planning to pull our piano back to Massachusetts on a trailer. While Jeff and I had lived out west for six years, his parents had provided a home for our plants and piano. This was the weekend we were to transport everything back to Gill. In my opinion, the US Mail seemed an adequate way of transporting the slides, but it wasn't fast enough for Jeff. Overnight mail was not a ready option in 1986. We would be stopping in New Haven on the way home.

We waved goodbye to the family in Chadds Ford on a sweltering Monday morning. Jeff's dad was still upright and strong, but a sadness hung about him and Muz as we left, and that feeling stayed with us as we rumbled out of the driveway. Jeff drove.

Once we had kids, Jeff and I started to negotiate over who won the right to drive on family trips. Driving involved constant attention to the road, to be sure, but the task was straightforward and relatively easy. When Jeff offered to drive, I was not fooled.

"Coin toss," I insisted, smiling but not joking. Tails, I lost. Being the passenger parent was hard work: crackers or peanut butter sandwiches and juice boxes for Willie, bottles of milk for the baby, cups of coffee from the thermos for the driver. The trip required almost nonstop entertainment by the non-driving parent. With me squeezed in the backseat between the kids' car seats, Willie and I read through the pile of picture books once, and then, by the time we turned onto Route 295 in New Jersey, we were going through them again. I wanted to read a new book Muz had given Willie that weekend, but he preferred reading and re-reading his favorites. I heard myself repeat the words aloud until my tongue twisted and my brain felt dry and shriveled.

As glad as I was to be with my little family, I found myself on edge when we were in the car together. Everything could go well. There were moments when we were all happy at the same time, but tranquility rarely lasted. Someone was bound to break down. We were dealing with heat, the kids, the dog, and the piano that loomed behind the car like a monster chasing us. Even scarier than a monster were the pathology slides that Jeff had tucked into the glove compartment. All of it added up to what portended to be a tense 330-mile trip.

After about an hour on the road, we drove up to a toll booth window at the entrance to the New Jersey Turnpike. Usually the toll-takers were notable only for their generic expressions, and we were just one of the multitude to pass by the ticket window. Jeff rolled down his window, and hot air blasted into the car. The ticket-taker stuck his head out from his booth and then stopped mid-reach as he took a long look at our car. From the front seat to the rear end, the station wagon was stuffed with gear. Then there was the trailer with a piano tied on with miles of rope and Jeff's Boy Scout knots. The guy leaned out over the booth, from the waist now, getting an eyeful of our traveling road show. Then he shouted to his buddy in the booth to our right.

"Hey, Joey!" he hollered, strong New Jersey accent even in those two words. "Looky what we got here. It's the Beverly Hillbillies! They're back!"

Joey looked through the window of his booth, saw our car and trailer, and cracked up at his friend's joke. I made myself as small as I could, shrinking between the two kids in the back seat, glad that I had not won the first driving stint after all. Jeff took the ticket when it was finally offered and stepped on the gas.

"Were they talking about us?" he asked as the window rolled up, silencing the laughter and insulating us from the smell of heat and automobile exhaust.

"I don't think they're used to seeing this kind of thing on the New Jersey Turnpike," I said. Neither of us had been feeling very lighthearted since leaving Chadds Ford, but when Jeff tilted the rearview mirror in order to see me, we both had to laugh at ourselves in the reflection.

The three o'clock deadline pressed on us, but we made good time, and I felt easier when we crossed the state line into Connecticut. At 2:45 we drove up in front of the Yale School of Medicine in New Haven and parked easily on a street that was deserted because of the holiday. First I felt relief at being there. Then I felt somber and sad. And hot. When Jeff disappeared into the building with the slides in his hand, I opened all the car doors so the kids, the dog, and I wouldn't melt inside. Getting the kids out of their car seats seemed too daunting a task in the heavy air.

In what seemed like a short time for such a serious mission, Jeff, empty-handed, appeared at the door of the building. He walked slowly back toward his carload of responsibility, not looking any lighter in spite of having handed over his burden. He poked his head into the car where we waited. Even with all of the doors opened, there was no air circulating around our sticky bodies. The three humans perspired, and the dog panted.

"He said he'll look over the slides tomorrow." He paused. Then he asked, as a kind of apology, "Do you want to go to the beach?"

We found our way to the waterfront in West Haven, a place where we had looked for each other on a Sunday afternoon nine years earlier in the days when we were just beginning to think we might want to get to know one another. But my mind did not linger over the past for very long. The parking lot was crowded, but Jeff found an empty spot, slipped the car into it, and shut off the engine. No longer a young couple on the edge of discovery, Jeff and I pulled ourselves and our charges out of the car. We were a sweaty and bedraggled bunch on a July afternoon, an unimaginable lifetime later.

BIRTHDAY

Late on the morning of July 12, a car occupied by four broadly smiling adults pulled into our driveway. The faces in the front seat belonged to my father and my Uncle Tommy, and in the back were my mother and her sister Ann. They thought they were coming to celebrate Willie's second birthday and Sarah's half-birthday. They had also been invited because we needed strong bodies to get the piano off the trailer, where it had been sitting since our return from Pennsylvania. What are relatives good for if not for moving furniture? Both sides of the extended family were always available for the modern equivalent of barn-raising, such as moving, house-painting, and garage-building. They arrived in good cheer with sleeves rolled up, prepared for the task at hand. The men wasted no time on social chitchat. They tolerated the greetings and then set out to inspect the piano where it sat on the trailer. Scratching their balding heads over the pluses and minuses of various moving options, the men circled the trailer to view the project from all directions.

In the middle of what had already been a hot summer, the day had dawned in an ominous shade of green-gray, and the sky doubled its threat as it reflected on the waters of Barton Cove. The air closed around us as the men eased the piano over the trailer's edge. I prayed that my father and uncle, who were fifty-something and former smokers, would not have heart attacks as they muscled the weight of the instrument across the stone walk and up to the narrow doorway that opened into the living room. While they sweated and occasionally swore, Willie played with curlicues of rainbow-colored ribbons dangling from a bouquet of balloons that floated along the dining room ceiling. My aunt and my mother passed Sarah back and forth while they took turns directing the men.

Saint Christopher, the patron saint of furniture movers, must have been watching over the men, because they experienced neither cardiac arrest nor lumbar strain, and the upright piano seemed to have come through its travels relatively unscathed, if completely out of tune. As Jeff settled the top of the piano into place, the air suddenly cooled and the breeze changed direction. With the moving done, it was time to start the party, and I made my way towards the kitchen to light the candles on Willie's birthday cake. Panting, Miss Weed pressed at my heels. I understood her anxiety when I heard the first rumbling in the distance, and then I saw a zigzag of lightning through a clearing in the trees. A few seconds later, thunder crashed over our heads, and the sky finally let loose its threat.

Over the noise of pounding rain and booming thunder, I called the group to the dining room table to sing the birthday song. The men wiped their foreheads with handkerchiefs and swallowed drinks from glasses dripping with condensation.

"Happy birthday to you . . ."

Everyone sang. I had every reason in the world to be happy. Willie was a fine two-year-old, Sarah was home, now smiling in the arms of her grandmother, and Jeff and I had seemingly jumped all of the hurdles required of us that year.

"Happy birthday to you . . . "

But in the week the piano had been languishing on the trailer, we learned that Jeff's dad did indeed have lymphoma—a non-Hodgkin's lymphoma that might not respond well to treatment—and would soon begin chemotherapy and radiation. I also felt some nagging, indefinable discomfort about Sarah. There was some worry that wouldn't leave me alone, an anxiety whose source I couldn't pinpoint.

"Happy birthday, dear Willie . . . "

Once the sky drained itself and the horizon cleared, it was time for folks to head home. Sunlight streaked across the yard as my dad backed the car from the curb and the sisters blew kisses.

"Happy birthday to you."

Jeff, Willie, and I waved goodbye to our visitors. Sarah rested in the crook of Jeff's arm. By all appearances, we were a privileged family with many reasons to be satisfied with our lives. Still, the ground felt uneven under my feet, and it would be some time before I could get used to trusting in our good fortune. Walking back to the house, I wondered how long it would take me to regain some confidence in my world.

CRISIS THEORY

In the years I spent caring for hospitalized patients who suffered through grave illnesses, I held onto the romantic notion that when a crisis occurred in a family, the individuals would band together and consequently draw closer to one another. I ought to have known better. On the medical floor at Yale-New Haven Hospital, I repeatedly saw patients and families who were traumatized by disease. Of course they rallied around their loved one when he or she was in the hospital. What I didn't think about was the day-in-and-day-out of living with a chronic or life-threatening condition.

In my first year as a nurse, I grew very fond of a patient I'll call Ellen. She was an elementary school teacher in her early thirties, and she had leukemia. Sometimes she was bald, sometimes she had a hint of peach fuzz on her head, but when she hadn't had a chemotherapy treatment for a long time and her hair grew in, it was a sassy red. She was married and had two darling, preschool boys, and the family was obviously tightly knit. To the twenty-one-year-old me, it seemed as if Ellen's life, previous to her illness, was like something out of a Norman Rockwell painting. Even when she was in the hospital, her life seemed very sweet. She had a caring husband and love and support from her family. When Ellen wasn't on precautions requiring visitors to wear gowns, masks, and gloves, the little boys came to see their mom. They giggled and played games and laid their heads in her lap while she stroked first the red hair, then the blond. Sometimes, when her husband came alone, the door to Ellen's room would be closed for a long time, and none of the nurses dared enter even when it was time to take Ellen's vital signs. They seemed like such a solid family. For a long time I didn't see clues indicating that the leukemia pervaded the family with as much destruction as it did Ellen's body.

In the last year of her life, Ellen was more comfortable in the hospital than she was at home. She had her own room on Winchester II, stayed in it for months at a time, and was an accepted part of the nurses' routine. "Who wants Ellen today?" was a standard question during the change-of-shift report. In fact, when she was away, I missed her. Room 1 was Ellen's room. It never felt quite right when some other patient was in there.

I didn't spend much time thinking about how Ellen's time away from her family might be a major stress on them. We, the nurses and doctors, were helping her stay alive with our fancy medical center treatments. I assumed the family would be grateful for that and happy she was alive even if she was living in the hospital. Then one day Ellen's husband pulled me aside to talk. The doctors had given Ellen permission to go home for a weekend between her treatments when her white blood cell count was high enough for her to safely leave the hospital, but Ellen told Michael she wasn't sure she wanted to go. She was afraid of getting an infection, she said. I could hear anger in Michael's voice, and I understood his frustration. We, the hospital staff, were now Ellen's family. She had come to a place where she was more comfortable with us and felt safer in the hospital than she did at home. The glow I had created around the picture of Ellen's family began to dissipate, and some understanding finally crept into my thinking. If this solid family struggled with love, loyalty, inertia, careers, time management, money, and daycare, then everyone must.

It wasn't until I experienced Sarah's birth that I internalized lessons I'd learned from Ellen's family. I found out the romanticized scenario of love and support I had pictured for others was a fairy tale I had clung to for too long, and the way the stress played out for Jeff and me was nothing like what I would have expected. We had to feel our way through the months when Sarah was in the hospital and even the months after her homecoming, like blind people, hands reaching forward to search for familiar landmarks, not recognizing unhealthy patterns as they slipped through our fingers.

I don't remember many scenes with Jeff that year except those that involved Sarah. I have more of a feeling about the atmosphere than pictures of him and me together. We didn't fight or argue. We functioned. When I look back at the year of Sarah's birth, I see a woman I hardly recognize and didn't like very much, then or now. I was so afraid of what might happen to Sarah that I hardened myself against feeling much of anything. I didn't cry very often. I tried to be light and cheerful with Willie, and I think I pulled that off well enough. But Jeff didn't get the benefit of my maternal playacting or my socially acceptable behavior to the hospital staff. Once Willie had gone to bed each evening, Jeff lived with an almost wordless wife. I got through the days. I cleaned the house, washed the dishes, folded the laundry.

Jeff went to the office every day, and the urgency of his work required attention and focus, allowing him to put aside worries about

Sarah and home for most of his ten to twelve hours away from home. He surfaced to find out how we were faring at some point each day, of course. He called me. He called the NICU. He talked to the neonatologists when there was something going on with Sarah and he wanted more details. I was out of the work force once Sarah was born, so I didn't have my professional self to fall back on. There was nothing to distract me from my worries. I had Willie to care for, but I often saw him as a liability—if he weren't so small and needy, I would be able to stay at the hospital for many more hours of each day. I thought being at the hospital all the time would be a good thing. I was depressed and I was afraid. My stomach hurt almost all the time.

I naïvely thought all would be well once Sarah came home, but as a family we were trading one set of stressors for another. Anyone who has added a new baby to the household knows the strain that comes with even a much-anticipated arrival to the family. Though we thought Sarah was finally well in the summer of 1986, the strain in our household had been above and beyond the norm for the six months preceding her discharge from the hospital, and that atmosphere had become chronic. It did not dissolve just because the baby came home. Stress continued to be present, but on an outpatient rather than an inpatient level of intensity.

While Jeff continued to be upbeat and optimistic about Sarah's progress that summer, I felt there were still reasons to fret. She seemed to be growing, but the pudgy look I had noticed over the Fourth of July weekend persisted. I found her appearance bothersome for some reason I couldn't articulate. Though she fed well most of the time, there were times when, without any warning or reason I could discern, she drank a bottle of formula and then suddenly blew the entire feeding across the room. It happened on an afternoon when we were visiting my mother.

Mom was taking care of Willie while Sarah and I went to the ophthalmologist to have her eyes checked. I had worried from the beginning about her vision, and I wondered what the doctor would say after the exam. I held her in my lap, my hand firmly on her forehead to keep her still while the doctor shined the bright light of the ophthalmoscope into the back of her eyes.

"Everything is normal," he said. "It is difficult to examine a baby at this age, of course, but her blood vessels look good. No signs of the proliferation of veins that can come with the high oxygen levels preemies need when their lungs are stiff. I think her vision will be fine."

I was happy and relieved when I delivered the news back at Grandma's. This was a big hurdle for Sarah. I sat on the sofa and fed her a bottle of her high-calorie formula and breast milk combination while I told my mother about the visit with the specialist. Sarah finished the bottle and then, without warning, she vomited explosively. There was milk all over the room. The violence of the vomiting brought on an episode of apnea. She still wore the apnea monitor when she was sleeping, but she hadn't experienced an episode of apnea in a long while. It was all too familiar. The color drained from her face, and her body suddenly became limp in my arms. I panicked momentarily. Then instinct kicked in, and I flipped her onto her abdomen to clear her mouth and jiggled her vigorously until she resumed breathing. I never got used to that feeling of suspended animation that happened during an apnea spell. It seemed like a very long time before she was breathing and her color was back to normal again.

The doctors couldn't give me an explanation for the vomiting. She did not have pyloric stenosis, a narrowing of the stomach where it leads to the small intestine. For the most part she kept her feedings down, but every now and then she would experience one of these episodes. Such events left me with a feeling of constant, low-grade unease.

Her hearing? She certainly turned and responded when we talked to her, so that seemed okay. Her breathing? Seemed normal except for the occasional apnea episode associated with those spells of vomiting. Her eyes? I worried about them until that mid-July visit. Still, I could always come up with a string of worries. Jeff was sure all would be well, but I couldn't get comfortable. I couldn't allow myself to be happy that today had been a good day. My eyes were always darting from side to side. I steeled myself for the next problem before it could sneak up on me.

There were two lectures I remembered best from my sophomore year in college. The very first lecture of my nursing career was entitled "The Hazards of Immobility." I can still visualize the title page of the journal article that accompanied the lecture: a pencil drawing of a patient in traction in a hospital bed. Until that time, I had no concept of how dangerous it was just to lie in bed.

The other lecture that stayed with me was called "Crisis Theory." The professor started the class by turning to the blackboard, where she drew a horizontal line with a piece of chalk. The straight line represented life she said, the uneventful times when an individual gets through the day the best way she can. She goes to work or school reliably, pays the monthly bills on time, has enough money for the necessities and maybe a little more, and has a reasonable support system of family and friends. The straight line indicated a time of balance and of general good health and well-being.

Then the professor drew a downward spike in the line, and that dip represented a calamity of some sort. The dip could be a deep one, like the upset caused by the death of a family member or a divorce after twenty years of marriage, or it could represent a smaller crisis like getting fired from a summer job at the local soft-serve ice cream bar. After the downward plunge, the line turned upward, indicating recovery from the crisis. At some point the line became horizontal and extended straight again. But here was the part that interested me. The professor drew two possible outcomes. In one, the line continued on the horizontal, but at a level that was higher than it had been before the dip that depicted the crisis. In scenario B, the other line came in at a lower level. I could see very clearly what she meant. Life continued after a crisis, but it was never the same as it had been. Whether a life was better or worse after a major event depended upon how the individual, couple, or family negotiated the dip.

Jeff and I had our ways of dealing with stress, some healthy and some probably not. Jeff's work day was long, and he didn't get much of a break when he walked into the house because by then I wanted to hand the kids over to him. I wasn't working. I stayed home with the kids and tried to assure myself this was the life I had been waiting for. But some indeterminate worry continued to gnaw at me. Name an organ system in Sarah's body, and I could recite a list of bad things that hadn't manifested themselves yet. We had worked ourselves into a pattern where Jeff was stuck carrying the burden of optimism while I lugged the worry. We traveled parallel lines, like two magnets of the same polarity with a force field keeping them apart. He couldn't express worry, knowing how antsy I was, and I wasn't able to be the strong one because he never let down his optimistic wall. If our lifeline was the one the nursing professor had used to illustrate her point, I suppose the line would have been on an upward trajectory in July. We were certainly moving away from the low point we had reached back in February when Sarah's daily reports were about weight loss, infection, malnutrition, heart murmur, and inadequate kidney function. Even so, it was a very slow climb back to where we'd started, and Jeff and I weren't blessed with much insight as we moved through the summer days. I knew things weren't quite right, but I didn't understand that we remained in crisis mode or that we were still working out a new horizontal level for our lifelines as individuals, as a couple, and as a family.

DUELING ANGELS

When I took Sarah for her weekly visit with our pediatrician at the end of July, he suggested it was time for her first immunizations.

"She weighs almost nine pounds and she's healthy," Hugh said. "It's time to get her started on her shots." Sarah was entering a new phase. We could actually begin to think of preventive health care for her.

An involuntary shiver ran through me at the thought of immunizations. I knew the fear was irrational, but it jumped up and bit me just as anything I perceived as a threat to Sarah was likely to do. When I worked in Wenatchee, new studies about the possible association between seizures and the pertussis vaccine were emerging, and research on that theory was still in progress. I had been skeptical of the connection at the time and preached to my patients that the effects of polio, diphtheria, pertussis, and tetanus were far more dangerous than any response to routine childhood vaccines might be. Nonetheless, in the week before Sarah's appointment for the injections, worry nagged at me.

Sarah received her vaccines on the first Friday of August, 1986. Even though I had given the same vaccinations to more babies than I could count, when it came to Sarah the process made me feel squeamish. I had always been confident when I reassured parents who hovered anxiously over their little ones. Now I was standing in everyone else's spot on the linoleum floor, suddenly suspicious of the doctor's word and the vaccines, and dreading the pain from the needle. I didn't want Sarah to experience any more pain.

The needle, syringe, and plastic vial of pink liquid appeared overly large as they lay on the stainless steel equipment tray. As Jean, the nurse, prepared to give the injections, I bent over the exam table and held both of Sarah's hands in one of mine and told her not to worry. It would be over quickly. Jean apologized to Sarah and carried on a steady stream of conversation while she squeezed the liquid into the corner of Sarah's mouth and then swabbed alcohol on the outside of her thigh. Sarah blinked when the needle plunged into the leg muscle, looked bewildered for a brief moment, but made no sound. It was over before I could let out my breath.

Two days later, Jeff stood at our pool's edge moving the vacuum slowly back and forth while Willie and I husked corn in anticipation of a backyard barbecue. We were looking forward to a visit from our Utah friends. David and Becky were visiting David's parents, who lived just an hour's ride from our home in Gill. They wanted to bring their parents along for the visit, and they especially wanted to introduce our babies to one another, for they had a young Sarah of their own.

After settling the arrangements for the weekend, I thought back to a night about two weeks after our Sarah had been born. It was around eight o'clock in the evening, and I clearly remembered the sound of the phone ringing and yawning blackness outside the curtainless kitchen windows. That was only our second January in Gill, and we were still adjusting to the economics of living in New England. We'd left relatively inexpensive electric heat back in Washington, but our drafty eastern house was being heated by an oil furnace that was almost as old as I was. The rooms never seemed warm enough or the lamps bright enough to counter the void of winter nights. I picked up the receiver, dreading what I might hear at the other end. Instead of a professional hospital voice, however, I heard David's mom.

"Becky wanted me to call you," she said, and I could hear the barely suppressed excitement in her voice. "They had a little girl last night. They named her Sarah."

I was thrilled for them. I called out to Jeff, "David and Becky had a baby girl!" He was happy, too. David and Becky had been waiting for the stork's arrival for some years. To their friends, who thought the couple eminently qualified to be parents, Becky's pregnancy seemed nothing less than a miracle.

"And how are you doing, Dear?" David's mom asked.

I wished I did not have to spoil the joy of her day with the gloom of our news. They didn't know our Sarah had been born. I wished I could tell her stories of cravings for pickles or swollen ankles or anything except what I had to tell. The tales were of two different Sarahs, infants at opposite ends of the country with birth stories as contrasting as the landscapes that separated them.

A few minutes after I ended my conversation with Mrs. Hall, the phone rang again. It was Becky this time.

"Why didn't you call me?" she asked with such concern in her voice that my own wobbled.

"I would have called you, but I didn't want to spoil the last weeks of your pregnancy," I told her. "I didn't want you to worry about your own baby."

"But Susan," she answered, "we can be happy about our baby and worried for yours at the same time."

I should have given them credit for that. Certainly they could feel both emotions simultaneously, but the birth of a first child is such an event that I had wanted their happiness to be pure. Of course life isn't like that, completely happy or completely sad. But I had not been able to bring myself to call them with news of a birth so radically different from the one they were anticipating, one I wanted them to have.

My mind had done this wandering as I pushed a cart through the grocery store and filled it with paper plates, cups, napkins, a watermelon for pool games, and chicken for the grill. I was looking forward to the reunion with our friends. At the same time, I was trying to squelch a niggling worry about Sarah. Normally she took a few naps during the day but had long periods of being awake, smiling, and taking part in family activities from wherever she might be perched. In the two days since her visit to the pediatrician, however, she had been sleeping more than usual, and when awake, she'd been fussy, which was very unusual for her. I thought she might be bothered by the immunizations and would sleep off the reaction after a few days. I added a bottle of liquid Tylenol to my cart. When I arrived home, I gave Sarah a few drops for the low-grade fever. I continued to make preparations for our guests, and between squeezing lemons and preparing the barbecue sauce, I watched her.

Standing at the top of a rise looking over our yard to the river, Jeff observed the scene before him. I walked over to join him. Unperturbed by sounds of play and conversation, Sarah slept in my arms. Our friends had arrived at around two in the afternoon, and it hadn't taken any time at all for us to share hugs and exchange kids. Armed with cold drinks and snacks, Jeff herded everyone into the back yard. Now he and I laughed as we watched David's father throw one Wiffleball after another to Willie, whose hands reached up with good intentions but invariably a few seconds after the ball had passed him by. From the comfort of a chair in the shade of a maple tree, David's mother observed her family with obvious contentment. Becky sat on a wooden swing that hung from that same tree while David stood with his feet spread and planted, pushing the swing. Becky had her arms firmly wrapped around the butterball in her lap. Their Sarah was a yellow-haired, peach-skinned, blue-eyed baby whose thighs bore secrets in their folds and whose cheeks dimpled with her toothy smile. Becky squealed loudly as she and her baby floated back and forth with David as their engine. Jeff draped one arm over my shoulders, and without taking his eyes from the tableau said, "Things might have been so different for us this year if we'd had them around."

I nodded. As we stood watching, I knew Jeff was saying that having such friends around would have lifted the burden from the two of us, even just a little. Jeff and I had been lonely for our far-flung friends in those first two years of living in Massachusetts. Maybe, if we had been in a different place or surrounded by the friends who were sprinkled around the country, the crisis of Sarah's birth would not have been so very hard.

We talked into the late evening in the low light of a living room that had not seemed so cozy in many months. In the worry and bustle of the time we'd been through, I hadn't allowed myself to dwell upon the absence of these friends and didn't realize how much I had missed them until we slipped into old camaraderie as if we were shuffling around in pairs of broken-in slippers. It was very satisfying to be with them and their robust baby.

The conversation faded into the background as I thought about how Sarah had taken almost nothing from her bottle all afternoon. With all the busyness of the barbecue behind us, I could no longer suppress the worry I felt as I held Sarah in my arms and we moved together forward and back in the rocking chair. She did not show any interest in drinking her formula or the Pedialyte I had found among my baby supplies. When I changed her diaper after what should have been her dinnertime, I noticed the faintest pink tinge around the edge of wetness from her urine. Huh, I thought, do the bright red Tylenol drops make the urine turn pink? I didn't think so. In the years of baby-sitting for kids, taking care of children in the hospital and, of course, changing Willie's diapers, a pink halo in the diaper was not something I had ever noticed. I grew increasingly distracted as the evening wore on. Earlier, I had given in to my private worry and told Jeff that Sarah wasn't acting like herself. From then on his attentions were divided by his role as the host, the parent for Willie, and co-worrier about Sarah, who had finally settled down in my arms. When the time neared nine o'clock, our friends gathered their belongings and said it was time to go.

Sarah slept through that night, which wasn't unusual for her, but it was a little surprising considering how fussy she'd been on the previous day. When she drank only an ounce from her bottle in the morning, and that only with much coaxing, Jeff and I agreed I should check in with Hugh when the office opened. I gave the receptionist five minutes to get settled with a cup of coffee for the Monday morning rush and picked up the phone to call the office at eight thirty-five. The woman who answered the phone said Hugh's appointments didn't start until one o'clock that day, and his schedule was full, but she could get us in at 5:15. Refusing to be alarmed, I did not insist on anything earlier. Yes, the baby was still a little feverish and not drinking very well, but the appointment was just so Hugh could pat me on the shoulder and tell me to quit being so nervous.

The hot day dragged. It should have been a typical Monday at home for Sarah, Willie, and me, but the hours felt anything but typical. After Willie's afternoon nap, we had some time to use up before the appointment, and I was too distracted to begin supper preparations. Thinking I'd allow our legs to carry us wherever the two-year-old would choose to go, I picked Sarah up from her cradle and followed Willie outdoors. Often there were places we were obliged to get to, so I was happy to give way to the sweltering afternoon and the open schedule and allowed Willie to blaze the trail.

We wandered according to his whim. Our property is a little less than two acres on the river's edge, but Willie chose the inland route, heading across the grass toward the woods. He was not interested in details. He didn't squat to find bugs or examine colorful rocks but seemed bent on putting as much distance as possible between himself and the house.

Willie toddled along on his own while I remained at a measured distance behind him with Sarah in my arms. She kept her eyes closed and seemed peaceful but too quiet. Usually she liked being outside. The sounds and smells interested and mellowed her. But on that day, whether we walked inside or out seemed to make no difference to her.

Something seemed to possess Willie as he ran down the hill onto the neighbor's property. Instead of wandering in aimless, distracted circles, as he normally would, he pushed farther away in search of something, though I couldn't guess what. After giving free reign to his curiosity for what I thought was a generous amount of time, I peeked at my watch from under Sarah's perspiring body and found it was already 4:30. Time to get back to the house.

"Come on, Willie!" I called to him. He did not turn, did not seem to hear. He did a little walk-run in the direction opposite of where I wanted him to turn, heading toward a water inlet that cut the neighbor's property in two. The depth of the water varied according to the opening and closing of the dam in Turners Falls below us and the reservoir at Northfield Mountain above us, but no matter what the level might be on that day, it was too deep for any child, and I didn't want him near it. He kept going.

"Willie!" I called to him in a cheerful, singsong voice that was supposed to cover my annoyance. "We have to go back to the house now." I didn't want to say, "Don't go too close to the water," because that would undoubtedly cause him to make a beeline for it.

He stopped just long enough to turn and look over his shoulder at me, and in that small motion I could see the gears of his mind working. I knew that he knew. He'd heard me the first time I'd called, and he understood that I wanted him to go back. It became clear to me that he was possessed at that moment by his terrible two-year-old urge to do exactly the opposite of what I was asking. Suddenly I was conscious of my heart beating in my chest. I felt the pulse in the back of my throat and the beginning of a roaring sound in my head. As if a switch had just flipped, my prevailing emotion suddenly changed from annoyance to fear.

When we were casually wandering the yard, I had allowed Willie a fifteen-foot lead, but now I stepped up my speed to catch up with him before he could reach the water. The inlet to the cove fell off abruptly from what was otherwise a flat lawn, and Willie would not even see the steep drop to the water until he was on top of it. I called to him again, "Willie, stop!" but he started to run, much faster than I thought he could. Wishing I didn't have to, but having no choice, I ran after him with the baby bouncing awkwardly in my arms. It felt wrong to accelerate without arms to help propel and balance me. I held the baby tighter. I needed to catch up with Willie. I needed to grab hold of some part of his body, kneel down in front of him, bring my face even with his round, Charlie Brown face, my eyes opposite his eyes and say, "Willie, we are going back to the house, now," and try to do it without clenching my teeth or losing my temper.

Running as fast as his long-for-his-age legs would carry him, Willie did not give me the chance to say anything. He was a long way from the house and maybe twenty feet from the water's edge. I ran too, trying not to jostle the baby too badly as I desperately hurried to keep the toddler out of the water. I asked myself, how are we going to get to the appointment on time? And then I wondered, how can I even get them safely back to the house?

When Willie was about ten feet from the water, I caught him by the back of his Winnie the Pooh shirt. The water was not really his destination, and it would certainly have added an element of surprise to his escapade. Growing up near the river had helped to make water a part of the landscape that was no more attractive to Willie than a dirt pile or a puddle in the driveway. But it was apparent he was simply trying to get as far away from me as he could at that moment, and he didn't care what was in his path.

I stood in that place, still holding the shirt while he squirmed, and tried to think through my options. Sweating, breathing hard, and simmering with a potentially explosive mixture of feelings, I bent over and awkwardly laid Sarah in the grass for a moment. I knew that while it might be August-dry, she would be safe and not going anywhere, unlike what her brother was trying to do. Her eyes were closed tightly as if in a theatrical sleep, and she did not fuss when I put her down.

Damn, I thought, between hard breaths and racing heartbeats, she doesn't even complain about the prickly grass.

I turned to Willie and squatted down. I placed my hands on his bony shoulders and glued my eyes to his. "Willie." I was looking into a red, sweating, furious face. "We have to go back to the house now. We need to get in the car and take Sarah to see Doctor Hugh." I didn't yell, but I emphasized every word.

"No!" he answered, turning to take off again. I grabbed a new handful of shirt.

I tried to explain to him. I knew that was a mistake even as I heard the words coming from my mouth, but I was still new to the art of parenting a child who could talk back to me. Willie had not shown such obstinacy in his short life. My choices were limited. I could not leave either one of them alone. He would run. She would be like a little Moses, a lonely baby asleep in the tall grass. I listened, wondering if I might shout for assistance from our neighbors. I didn't hear any engine noise at the moment, but Al or Lea could come around a corner and drive by on a lawnmower or a tractor and not even see a baby on the grass. I looked around but it was apparent I wouldn't find any help from their direction. A retired couple, they were nearly always working in their gardens but were likely to be making supper preparations at this hour, and the house was more than a holler away.

Though my hand was nowhere near his neck, Willie was making strangled noises and squirmed under my grasp. He threw himself down and flopped on the grass like a hooked fish. He was nearly as slippery. He refused to walk. Finally, frantic and with no other choice, I stood over Willie and immobilized him between my ankles. Somehow, I bent over sideways without losing my balance and gathered Sarah into one arm in the football hold I had learned in my pediatric nurse years—her bottom squeezed between my right elbow and hip, her head supported in my right hand. With my stronger left arm, I then scooped the recalcitrant toddler up to my left hip and hoisted him into a secure, if uncomfortable, hold.

Until that moment, I'd had few occasions when I had to push myself to the limits of physical ability. Dragging myself, panting, over the rocky scree at the top of a Yellowstone mountain came to mind. But there I was, on a ninety-degree afternoon in August in a challenging physical situation I had never anticipated. Willie, the little boy who was just finding out who he was, did not want to change direction, and he proceeded to throw a mighty fit, howling with lung-clearing bursts of pre-verbal profanity. Garnering every bit of strength, I carried the quiet baby ever so gently on my right side while employing a vice grip on the thirty-pound fury I carried on my left. It was if I had a gentle angel swathed in white gossamer sitting on my right shoulder, guiding me as I carried a glass ornament, and a pit bull with wings on my left who took the cigar out of his mouth only to say, "Yeah! Yeah! You can do it, Lady. Don't let go, no matta what." Willie writhed and twisted and screamed over the fifty-yard hike up the hill to the driveway. I prayed I would not damage either one of them.

The station wagon was parked on the driveway in the shade of a tall pine. Before starting our walk, I had moved the car out of the sun and opened the windows so the heat wouldn't smother us when we got in. When I set the struggling Willie down on the driveway, he ran again, so I quickly slipped the still-quiet baby through the open window on the passenger side of the car. Grateful she still was not able to roll over, I carefully laid her down on the back seat and then turned to chase Willie down once more. As I caught up to him, scooped him up, and lugged him back to the car, I saw what a mess he was.

Oh, Lord, I thought. It isn't supposed to be this way. In order to put Willie in the car seat, I first had to get him to bend at the waist, and then I strapped him in, a furious, sweaty, crying little boy, his face streaky with angry tears, his shirt showing evidence of everything he'd eaten that day, his hands unmentionable. Without the fifteen minutes I had anticipated for getting us ready before the appointment, the office visit had become a come-as-you-are affair.

I turned my attention to Sarah, whose eyes were open but not showing any sign of upset in response to the noise surrounding her. In contrast to the aerobic running and weight lifting I'd just done with Willie, I picked the baby up as if I were dancing in a ballet, my arms soft as I gentled her nine-pound body into her infant seat. And I used to wonder that children from the same two parents can turn out so differently, I thought.

I turned the car's air conditioning on high as we headed out of the driveway. My hair was flattened with sweat and clinging to my forehead, and my tee shirt stuck to my chest and back. Sarah lay in her seat, oblivious to the commotion, her eyes closed again as if she were listening to a lullaby instead of a screaming brother. They are going to take both of them away from me when they see us like this, I thought. I am a basket-case-failure-wreck-of-a-mother.

Willie quieted down by the time we arrived at the office parking lot, and when I opened his door and unbuckled his seat belt, he eased one leg and then another out of the car as if we were on a normal afternoon outing. With complete composure, he walked into the building, even placing his sticky hand in mine as we crossed the lot. Once in the office, he let go of my hand and calmly went over to the PacMan game that didn't need quarters. I had some baby wipes in the diaper bag I was carrying and considered using one to remove some of the grime stuck to Willie's skin but decided it wasn't worth disturbing the peace. I did, however, take the opportunity to wipe off my own hands. A happy-if-dirty little guy, Willie was content to sit in a chair that was just his size where he could push buttons and make the little men do what he commanded them to do. He had spent all his energy for his personal re-sistance movement that afternoon and was ready to be the perfect child.

In awe of the behavior shift, I watched him for a minute. Then I moved to stand in line before the receptionist's window. Sarah slept in my arms.

In the exam room, I took Hugh through the events of Sarah's weekend. He listened, pensive, not interrupting while he kept his eyes on the baby. She didn't fuss as she lay on the exam table. Hugh took his stethoscope from around his neck. He bent over Sarah and listened to her heart, lungs, and abdomen. He removed the stethoscope from his ears and I told him of another strange thing that had happened after our guests departed the evening before. When I removed Sarah's diaper, an unnecessary exercise since it was hardly wet that day, not only had I noticed the pink tinge once again, but I also saw a weird, fibrous glob sitting on the surface of the diaper. I had never seen anything like it. It wasn't stool, I was certain. It was tan and not slimy, as I would have expected, but stringy.

Hugh moved his hand gently over Sarah's belly and palpated under her ribs on the right to feel her liver, then on the left to feel her spleen in that knowing, doctor's way. I pulled a plastic sandwich bag out of my diaper bag and handed it to Jean, the nurse who had weighed Sarah on this day just as she had the previous Friday. Hugh lay Sarah back on the table and then took the Baggie and manipulated the glob through the plastic. He managed to keep his face impassive, accustomed, I imagined, to the strange things kids inserted into and eliminated from their bodies. But he, too, was mystified by this one.

"Let's send that to the lab," he said to Jean and handed the Baggie back to her.

He was puzzled by Sarah's illness. What I found most alarming was that he did not think her symptoms were due to the immunizations.

"What do you mean?" I asked, a terrible dread grabbing like a claw at my chest. "What else could it be?"

"I don't know," he answered honestly. "We'll get some blood work, a urinalysis, and some cultures." Jean gathered a small catheter to obtain a urine sample as well as a tourniquet and alcohol swabs and butterfly for blood drawing. Somehow Hugh managed to find a vein in Sarah's arm to draw the blood. She hardly flinched as the needle entered her skin, and that was more frightening than anything that had happened all afternoon. It was one thing for Sarah to sleep through Willie's tantrum. It was another for her to be unresponsive to a needle being stuck into her arm.

Hugh said, "I'll call you with the results as soon as I get them. Get her to drink as much as you can through the night."

Jeff was just getting out of his car when we returned home. He walked up to my window, and I rolled it down. He looked at me and then past me, and his eyes ran over what must have looked like a God-awful mess of a family. He knew where to start and opened the door next to Willie. The cheerful little boy said, "Hi, Daddy," and allowed himself to be released from his car seat and scooped into his dad's arms.

Jeff carried Willie into the house, and I unhitched Sarah from her seat and followed the guys. I doled out the details to Jeff as we made our way through supper and baths. We all needed to sleep off the day and prepare for the next.

That night I felt as if we were on an airplane in a holding pattern, circling in the air. I saw our destination far below but was unable to land. Jeff went to work early the next morning, and I waited to hear from Hugh. The kids and I followed the normal routine, and I heard myself talking to Willie in a fake happy voice. When the phone rang mid-morning, I didn't want to answer it as if hearing the news could start our circling airplane on a downward plunge with nothing but gravity in control. I picked up the receiver. It was Hugh.

"She has yeast in her urine," the pediatrician said matter-of-factly.

"Yeast?" I asked. "What do you mean, yeast?"

"I don't know yet," he answered. "I've scheduled her for an ultrasound at Baystate tomorrow morning at ten. We could do it here, but they have her old records there. The right people can look at it while you're down there, instead of you having to wait for a report."

I appreciated Hugh's thoroughness, but the fact that the procedure would be the very next day seemed both a relief and a bad omen. It wasn't easy to schedule an ultrasound so quickly. He must be worried.

"Thank you, Hugh. We'll be there."

I sat down, looking at the telephone receiver in my hand. The steady buzz of the disconnected line sang on. Gently, I placed it back in its cradle and continued to hold my hand on it. Then I picked up the receiver once again and punched in the numbers to Jeff's beeper.

ALL DRESSED UP AND NO PLACE TO GO

At 9:50 on the following morning, I sat outside the ultrasound room at Baystate Medical Center. Sarah slept in my arms. On my way out of town I had taken Willie to Lynda's. He'd walked one by one up the steps to her kitchen, each foot meeting the other on the tread before going to the next. His swimsuit and towel were folded into his Sesame Street backpack. Jeff didn't come with Sarah and me to Baystate. He had a schedule full of patients, and there was no need for both of us to spend the morning in waiting rooms.

This particular waiting room was stark, and the chairs were not the cushy kind one expects to find in a medical office. I was put off by its ascetic atmosphere until I realized it was probably a holding room for in-patients. There was little furniture in order to leave space for those who were wheeled into the room in wheelchairs or on gurneys. The room wasn't set up for patients who would arrive under their own power to sit anxiously on the edge of the straight-backed seats.

Sarah was still very quiet, dressed on that morning as if for a party. In the months after her birth, friends sent her presents when they perceived that the news from the hospital was a little bit hopeful. On this day, I dressed her in one of those gifts, a white dress with pale, multi-colored threads embroidered in a pattern on the front smocking. A pair of white panties, all puckered and ballooned, matched the dress and completed the outfit. The dress fit her nine pounds perfectly though I thought it impossible that her thighs would ever fill out the elastic circumference on the panty legs. I did not dress her up very often, but this seemed like a special occasion in an odd sort of way. I remembered from having Willie that if we did not use an outfit when it fit, he might pass right through the size within a few weeks and never be able to wear it. What was I thinking? That was Willie, the kid born in the ninety-fifth percentile for length, who grew out of his pajama bottoms overnight. Here lay Sarah, who, at eight months of age, still hadn't reached ten pounds. She might be wearing the same outfits for a year.

The technologist called us in, and I began to undress Sarah on the exam table quietly to match her quiet, but she did not protest at the inter-ruption of her sleep or the cold of the room or the hardness of the table. I held her body in one hand and unbuttoned and slid the dress over her head with the other. Sarah had developed what the doctors called col-lateral circulation to compensate for her earlier IV placements. There were new veins between her neck and right shoulder. The tangle of blue veins that showed from under the skin above her shoulder seemed more prominent in the fluorescent light. She is going to hate us for these flaws when she grows up, I thought. I hoped. I traced the veins as I often did when she was undressed, and her skin was warm and soft under my fingertips. I left her socks on; there was no harm in that. When she was down to just a diaper and white socks, I laid her on the table. I moved around to the opposite side and out of the way while the technologist finished setting up the machine and then darkened the room.

The quiet seemed unnatural. We were in an oasis of silence in the midst of the chaos of a medical center that probably employed as many people as live in the town of Gill. I stroked Sarah's head, her hair fine and close. My finger circled the spongy, cherry-red hemangioma that still dotted her forehead at the hairline. It was shrinking but still there, a little smaller than a dime. She reflexively curled the fingers of her left hand around my index finger while the technologist applied a clear gel to her belly and back. She did not protest. He left her on her back and worked the transducer over her body. He slid it around her abdomen with his right hand and lifted her body with his left in order to reach around to her back. His eyes remained fixed on a video screen that sat on a portable table.

A sliver of light flashed on the wall, and I could hear the door close behind me. The physician. While the tech did his work, the doctor introduced herself in church-like tones as Barbara Stechenberg. She said she was from the division of infectious disease. She had consulted on Sarah when she'd had her fungus infection during the winter and had followed Sarah's progress through her hospitalization.

Dr. Stechenberg shifted her attention up to the screen and moved closer to get a better look. Pointing to the shadows on the screen, the doctor and technologist discussed the ultrasound in a language I couldn't translate. I understood the words they were saying, but I didn't know whether in the end they would tell me the findings were normal or pathological. No surprise registered in their voices, and I allowed myself to feel reassured by the absence of alarm in their conversation.

The technologist turned the lights on.

"You can get Sarah dressed," Dr. Stechenberg said to me, "and I will be right back to talk to you."

I slipped the white puff over Sarah's head. After inserting a little arm into each sleeve, I turned her over gently and buttoned the back of the dress. She didn't fuss. Her eyes were open but her world was still very small, and she didn't register much beyond the person who was in her immediate presence. I found her diaper and looked at it closely. Dry. The tabs were still sticky, so I could use it again. Diaper on. Pantaloons over the diaper. Tiny white booties on her stockinged feet. Passive, she allowed me to do whatever I wanted. I rubbed her bare legs to reassure myself of her presence as much as to warm her.

The doctor returned, filling the room with her authority.

"It looks as if Sarah may have fungus in both of her kidneys," Dr. Stechenberg told me directly, but not unsympathetically. She was an *A* physician in the imaginary book I had filed months before on a shelf way back in my mind. "Most likely it is a recurrence of the fungus ball she developed as a newborn. Sometimes this happens. Fungus walls itself off so effectively that even weeks of medication cannot get to it. Both of her kidneys are full."

I remember looking at the doctor, my ears ringing. I was thinking how nice it was she could take the time to come down here, to this room, to talk to me in this way, so directly, when she was probably very busy that day, and we hadn't been on her schedule. When she stopped talking, explaining, and I caught up to her words, I could not quite grasp what they meant. Her voice was calm as she said terrible things. Frightening words that didn't fit. It was like having the wrong soundtrack on a movie.

"We'll have to admit Sarah to the pediatric floor," she finally said, clarifying what should have been obvious to me.

I experienced what felt like the neurological equivalent of a cardiac arrest. A brain arrest. I stopped thinking. The air in my lungs hung suspended, not moving in or out. What was I expecting? I had dressed Sarah up as if she were going to the county fair with the hope that if she looked adorable she would win the blue ribbon of good health and then go home with a prize. In spite of the worry I had struggled against all weekend, I had deluded myself on the silent ride in the car to Springfield that she would have a test, there would be an answer, and there would be a treatment. I had not allowed myself the thought that the hospital would keep her or that she might not be in the car with me on the ride home.

The doctor left to make preparations for Sarah's admission to the pediatric unit, and I looked at my baby. Her eyes were closed. She lay fully dressed in what now seemed like a ridiculous outfit. I felt betrayed. I was aware of what an odd reaction that was, and I felt ashamed. But it seemed as if Sarah had been holding out on me. She falsely posed as a well baby when, in truth, she was harboring disease, fungus balls bursting like fireworks on the Fourth of July and broadcasting their prolific spores through her kidneys. This illness had developed in front of my eyes every day while I washed, changed, fed, and played with her.

Half sentences and partially formed thoughts tumbled in my brain. Part of me wondered, how will this baby, this sweet, precious, vulnerable baby, get through this new invasion . . . ? Mixed up with that thought was the end of the sentence . . . and how will I?

On the day we discovered Sarah had the fungus infection in her kidneys, I stayed with her at the hospital until about nine in the evening. Her ultrasound had lasted only about a half hour that morning, but it took until the early afternoon for a room to open up on the pediatrics floor. I spent the afternoon being interviewed about Sarah's medical history by both an intern and a medical student. By five o'clock Sarah was in a crib in her new room, and I was holding her in position while one of the doctors performed a lumbar puncture to rule out infection in the spinal fluid. Then the nurses set about starting an IV and began her first therapy with amphotericin b, the dreadful medication she'd received while in the NICU. It all seemed terribly familiar.

I had called Lynda when it became apparent the day was falling apart, and she kindly agreed to keep Willie for as long as necessary. I had also interrupted Jeff at the office with the news. He and I did not always interpret Sarah's medical problems with the same sense of alarm, but when I told my husband, the kidney doctor, what they'd found on ultrasound, I heard only silence at the other end of the phone. I knew at that moment we were in deep trouble.

It felt eerie to be back in the old routine as if June and July had been the aberration: Jeff to work, Willie to Lynda's, Susan back and forth from the hospital, Sarah in the hospital. I spent the week walking around with a weird kind of drug-high feeling. We were still circling in that airplane. Though there had been a big drop in altitude, we had leveled off. There was something oddly reassuring in having a diagnosis, I guess, because after the undefined worry about her lethargy, lack of appetite, pink urine, and the weird glob in her diaper, the candida infection was something familiar. It was a devil I knew instead of one I hadn't met before.

The plan was straightforward, and I was already familiar with that as well. Sarah would begin a ten-week course of two medications: amphotericin b was to be administered intravenously while another medicine 5-fluorocytosine was given orally until the fungus in both kidneys was eradicated. I couldn't process, yet, how long that would be. I couldn't allow myself to picture life at home without her. Dr. Stechenberg had even mentioned that once Sarah's treatment regimen was set, she might be transferred to the Franklin Medical Center. I was too distracted to pay attention to "maybes" and didn't ask when that might be. All I knew was when I went to see Sarah each day, even though she wasn't her bright-eyed self and her skin was a pasty hue, she was alert enough to know me. By the end of the week, she actually smiled a greeting. Sarah had started to smile that summer but had lost her smile when she'd become sick. I was happy to see her toothless grin again.

She was in a room by herself. We decorated her crib with a mobile that dangled from above. The singing yellow bird she'd had in the NICU sat in one corner of the crib. Lammy (now known as Yammy per Willie's prounnunciation) came too. Lammy was much quieter in the hospital than he had been at home with Willie ringing his bell in Sarah's face.

As the week went on, I continued to feel anxious but a little manic, overly cheerful with a matter-of-fact, this-too-will-pass kind of optimism. I wasn't afflicted with the same sense of despair I'd had after Sarah was born because she was so much different from the premature newborn she'd been in the winter. There was so much more to her. She weighed nine pounds. Though her color wasn't good, her face and cheeks were full. Sometimes she was fussy, especially when the medicine started giving her diarrhea and she had frequent, loose stools that made her bottom red and sore. But often she was social, and her eyes followed the mobile or turned toward the tinny music that the yellow bird played when its string was pulled.

The IV pump sat by her crib with an aluminum foil snake extending from the bag of medicine just like in the old days. The doctors had two major concerns: abnormal lab values indicated Sarah's kidney function was suffering as a result of the infection, and she had precious few veins for IV's. She would need intravenous therapy for almost three months, and it quickly became apparent she wouldn't have enough superficial veins to use for IV's. On the evening of her admission, someone found a vein in her scalp above one ear. It was a ridiculous place for an IV. I watched a nurse hang the first dose of medication scheduled to run in over four hours. I knew the fragile IV site wouldn't last much beyond that. By the time she needed her treatment the next day, the scalp IV had blown, and she needed to have a new one inserted.

Blood drawing was a nightmare. There were no veins in her arms. She had a small vein in one hand. Once I walked in to find an IV poking out from her ankle at an precarious angle. She needed a central IV line, and soon.

To complicate things further, Sarah's blood cultures showed that the candida was in her blood as well as her kidneys. Once they knew that, the doctors said they couldn't put a central line into a vein while her blood was infected. So it was a Catch-22: she needed the IV medicine in order to clear the infection, and she needed veins in order to get the medication in.

Though she made friends with the doctors, nurses, and other staff, Sarah was often alone. I felt uncomfortable with the thought that she spent lots of time awake and by herself. Babies shouldn't be alone. They need words and music to listen to and faces to smile at and interact with. Sarah was rarely alone at home except to sleep. I couldn't blame the nurses for the lack of staff, but what could I do? The time struggle hadn't changed, and we were in our old dilemma. Sarah looked okay, and I had to hope and trust she received enough attention over the course of a day. I marked off the days on the calendar one by one. We would get through this.

Two days before Sarah was readmitted to the hospital, I'd taken her and Miss Weed for a ride in the car. I'd waited for a time when Willie was at Lynda's. Willie's tolerance for errands was minimal while the baby and the dog were quiet and faithful company. I drove to Leyden, a small hill town about ten miles from Gill, to buy fresh-picked wild blueberries. I had made jam the previous summer, and I planned to do that again. Mostly, though, I loved bringing the berries home and eating as many as I wanted.

After Sarah went into the hospital, the cardboard box sitting on the countertop loomed over the room. It haunted me when I was in the kitchen. I avoided looking at it. I didn't know what to do with all of those berries. The memory of a sweet drive on a summer day with my baby sleeping in the car seat was now tainted, and the box seemed to taunt me with the innocence or ignorance it represented. I was standing in the kitchen, feeling overwhelmed by berries and a life that had become so complicated, when I heard a knock on the door and a "Hello?" One of the counselors from family planning had called a little earlier to see if she could stop by. Barbara and I worked together only one afternoon each week, but in the nine months of our acquaintance, I had developed great respect for the way she did her work.

We stood at the kitchen counter and talked about Sarah. Then, with her counseling skills fully engaged, Barbara looked at me directly. "How are you, Susan?"

I shrugged my shoulders. How I might be feeling seemed obvious. Why would I want to run through the litany?

Then she asked, "Are you seeing anyone?"

At first I didn't know what she meant. That was a question I would pose to my single friends.

"Oh." I got it. "You mean a therapist?"

She nodded.

"No. Why would I need a therapist?"

She half smiled. "Have you ever worked with a therapist?"

I never had. In my previous life I had considered myself a pretty together person. I'd never had a reason to seek counseling. The thought hadn't occurred to me.

"Why would I need a therapist?" I repeated. It seemed reasonable for me to feel scared, anxious, depressed, worried, and tired. I was reacting the way I would expect anyone should react under the circumstances. How could a therapist help with that?

Barbara persisted, asking the right questions, and she let me hear my own answers. She left me with a hug and also with a name and phone number scribbled on a piece of paper.

Considering how short Barbara's visit was, I was surprised to find the kitchen didn't seem so gloomy after she left. Then, for some reason, I walked over to the counter where the cardboard box sat. I picked up the box and carried it out to the garage where I had an upright freezer. I opened the freezer door, moved everything around to clear a shelf, and shoved the box in. I slammed the freezer door behind me, walked back into the house, and stopped worrying about what I should do with ten pounds of blueberries.

The truth was, in that first week, my varying responses to Sarah's return to the hospital had morphed into a hyperpositive frame of mind. My newfound attitude came out of a cheerleader-like sense that we could manage this crisis. Sarah has an infection, I told myself and then started to rationalize. She's had it before, and it went away. She'll get better again.

I was also obsessing about our family vacation plans. We were supposed to start our vacation on August 10. We had planned to spend a week at my parents' summer house in Falmouth, on Cape Cod, and two families who had been our friends since our Yellowstone days were joining us. Jay and Kim were planning to drive up from Durham, North Carolina, with their daughter. Jim and Eileen were flying from Grand

Junction, Colorado, with their two children. As a group, our children ranged in age from seven-month-old Sarah to four-year-old Nathaniel. Jeff and I were looking forward to a week of catching up with buddies who had moved from being singles to being married with children, just as we had done. We were really anticipating the week, and I was doubly disappointed that the onset of Sarah's new illness changed all of that.

Jay was the ambulance driver / cook / maintenance man at the Yellowstone Hospital during our summers there, and Kim X-rayed the kidney stones and broken bones tourists suffered while vacationing in the park. Jim and Jeff had shared a dormitory room ten years earlier in Gallup, New Mexico, where the two internists had brushed up on their baby-delivering skills in fulfillment of two-year commitments each of them had made to the Indian Health Service. Eileen was a nurse and also a Yellowstone friend, and Jeff took credit for the matchmaking that had resulted in their marriage.

A Cape Cod vacation seemed ideal. The five little kids would mix and match on the beach and in the water. I envisioned days with adults helping their sun-screened children build sand castles at the ocean's edge and evenings spent eating sumptuous meals of fresh fish and clams. When the kids were asleep, we would play board games late into the night. We could spend the week figuring out how we had managed to travel down the road from Yellowstone's adult summer camp and dormitory life to a time when we had six careers, three houses, and five kids among us.

On August 6 when I called Eileen in Colorado to tell her about Sarah's hospital admission, she murmured sympathetically and assured me they could make other plans. I could not bear the words, my heart shriveling at the thought of not seeing these people. I remembered how rejuvenating the afternoon with David and Becky had been. I needed our friends more than ever.

I shamelessly begged Eileen on the phone. My words ran together because I didn't want to leave any gaps when she might say no.

"Please come, please, please, please come. You already have the time scheduled. We have the pool, we have the river. We can play just as well here as we can at the Cape. We can eat fish and lobsters. We have a blender, and we can make strawberry daiquiris. I picked the strawberries myself in June and froze them. The kids won't know they aren't at Cape Cod. Each day, one of you can come with me to the hospital. Jim and Jeff can go together later. You can see the baby and keep me company. The rest can stay and play with the kids. I want you to see her. She is so precious, and you will love her. I want you to know her. Please, please come."

Eileen protested from Grand Junction. Jay protested from Durham. They thought we had too many worries, and they would be too much trouble. But the desperation in my voice must have traveled. When the circle of phone calls had been completed—Gill to Durham, Durham to Grand Junction, and Grand Junction to Gill—the plan was settled. After mulling over the options, the two couples decided they would come to scenic Gill, Massachusetts, for their summer vacation.

I was hugely relieved as if they were rescuing me from a brink or an edge I couldn't see.

Jeff and I set about making preparations. We put sheets on the pull-out sofa and the bed in the guest room. He dragged sleeping bags from closets. I filled the refrigerator. On Sunday afternoon, right on schedule, a rental car pulled into the driveway, and the Colorado family poured out. Within fifteen minutes they had spilled open the contents of their suitcases. Nathaniel and Adrienne tossed aside shorts, tee shirts, and sandals, wriggled into swimsuits, ran outside, and jumped into the pool. Trusting souls, they hadn't even stopped to test the temperature of the water. I hadn't even offered anyone cold drinks. Willie stood by the pool, transfixed, not sure about the whirlwind that had just swept through his house.

Later, a car bearing North Carolina plates crossed the Massachusetts border as the sun was dropping behind the Connecticut River. On the ride up Route 91, Jay and Kim recognized the sign for Baystate Medical Center and decided to drive off Exit 10 in Springfield to search for Sarah on the pediatric floor. They took turns visiting with her as she lay in her crib, one of them staying in the waiting area with their little girl, Canden. Then Jay called from the pediatrics floor at the hospital.

"Hey, there." I recognized the Blue Ridge Mountains in the two words. "This here little gal is lookin' pretty damned good." A southern gentleman, Jay always has a compliment for the ladies. I had seen Sarah that morning, and she'd looked double chinned and sallow. But she was more pleasant than she had been since her admission to the hospital six days before and was gratifyingly alert as she reclined in the infant seat that allowed her to sit up in her crib.

"Give her a kiss good night for all of us, and get yourselves up here," I said to Jay, my own voice waxing a little twangy under his influence.

"All right. We'll be headin' on up real soon."

I hung up the phone and went into the kitchen to report to the others. We dressed the kids in their pajamas, and the three of them went out to chase lightning bugs in the back yard. By the time the dark fully settled in, the mosquitoes had made themselves more annoying than the lightning bugs were fun, and everyone returned to the house. The doorbell rang, and I heard, "Hey! Is anybody home?" All at once, the house was full of more suitcases, more hugs, and lots of southern comfort.

TESTS OF MANHOOD

Three days later, everyone at the Gill resort was outdoors taking advantage of a perfect August afternoon. This was Sarah's eighth day in the hospital. On the previous day, Tuesday, Eileen had come to the hospital with me. When we walked into Sarah's room, she was awake, sitting upright in her infant seat with her mobile turning a slow rotation in front of her eyes. She looked peaked, but she smiled when she saw me. Or maybe it was Eileen she smiled at because everyone smiles when Eileen enters a room. Even so, while Eileen fussed over Sarah, I stood momentarily rooted to the floor. The right side of Sarah's face and neck was puffy and distorted, and it took me a moment to understand what I was seeing. Before I had a chance to call for a nurse, one walked in.

"Why is her face so swollen?" I asked though I knew even as the words came out. There was only one explanation.

The nurse seemed apologetic. The IV that had been placed in a vein in Sarah's scalp the night before had infiltrated. That one fragile vein had been all they could find in their desperate search for a place to insert the IV, but it hadn't been sturdy enough to withstand the volume of fluid and caustic medication flowing into it. Fluids had seeped into surrounding tissues for some time before anyone had noticed the vein wasn't working. Sarah smiled again when I went over to her crib to pick her up, but it was a crooked, wan smile that made me want to cry rather than smile back.

Her appetite had not improved since her admission to the hospital. When I tried to feed her, she would take very little from the bottle before pushing the nipple out of her mouth. She did no better with the nurses. The doctors ordered increased thickness in her formula to boost the calories, but she wasn't much interested. To complicate the picture, she was also having frequent, seedy, green stools as a side effect of the medications. Her abdomen was distended, and she often made grunting sounds when she breathed. She looked and sounded uncomfortable even as she attempted to be cheery.

On that sunny afternoon when the rest of us were playing by the pool, Sarah was scheduled for an ultrasound of her kidneys. I stayed home while Sarah was having the procedure and planned to go to the hospital that evening.

At three o'clock the kids woke from their naps. They all ran outside to frolic between the yard and pool with adults who'd grown childlike themselves as the responsibilities of work grew more remote. That afternoon the fathers were performing "tests of manhood" per Jeff's rules. The first test required heaving a tennis ball over, not into, the treetops that filled the yard beyond which the waters of Barton Cove glinted in the afternoon sun. The oaks and maples were mature, and their leafy branches reached high and wide. The ball had to fly over the trees and land with a plop in the river; a shoreline thud did not earn the thrower the manly title or the beer that went with it. The game had entertained them for much of the day though some of the contestants never accomplished anything more than keeping Miss Weed busy as she retrieved failed attempts.

After the ball-throwing contest, the swimming pool became the venue for the tube jump event. Jeff continued as program director for another hour of activities.

By five o'clock, the kitchen was overflowing with water-wrinkled children and sun-tired parents getting a start on happy hour and making preparations for the junior dinner seating. The phone rang. Eileen was closest and grabbed it.

"Blomstedt-LaScala Summer Resort," she answered, suppressing the laugh she had been ready to let loose. I watched to see if the call was for Jeff or me, and her face changed.

"Yes, she's right here." She covered the receiver with her hand and almost whispered, "Susan, it's the hospital." Shushing everyone, she handed the phone to me. "It's the hospital," she said again to the room, and everyone grew quiet, their eyes glued to my face.

"Hello, Mrs. Blomstedt, this is [a name I didn't recognize] at the pediatric intensive care unit," said the voice in my ear. It was a small voice and sounded very far away. I didn't catch the name, but the voice went on. "Sarah . . . ultrasound today . . . central line . . . a seizure." I pressed my finger over the ear not attached to the phone as I stretched the cord as far as it would go into the next room. I thought I wasn't hearing right.

"What?" I said. "I'm sorry. I really couldn't hear you."

The voice said more distinctly, "The baby had her central line put in yesterday." I knew that. On Saturday Jeff and I had gone to see Sarah, and the doctors said Sarah had no more veins for IVs. We had signed a permit for her to go to the operating room sometime in the next few days in order to have a catheter inserted into a large vein near her heart. That vein, like a large river, could tolerate having extra fluids and medications flow into it. Once the central line was in place, there would be no more painful IV insertions. Sarah's blood had to be clear of candida before they could do the surgery, so the doctors had been waiting for negative blood cultures before they could go ahead. Finally on Tuesday, they had taken her to the operating room and surgically inserted the line.

The voice went on with its painstaking explanation. "She went to ultrasound this afternoon to recheck her kidneys. When she got back to the floor, she had a seizure. She's been moved to the pediatric ICU. She's intubated, on a respirator." And then he said the words I'd never heard before, "You'd better come."

You'd better come. The call we had dreaded for the first three months of her life came on a summer day when I'd let down my guard, when I had never given a thought to such a possibility. I found my way back into the kitchen and placed the receiver back on its cradle. I turned to the room and said to the adults, "Sarah's had a seizure. They don't know why. She's in the pediatric ICU." Feeling lost, I paused for a minute. I wasn't sure what to do next. Then I said, "I have to go out and tell Jeff."

The happy noises of dinner preparations stopped. Sounds of ice tinkling in glasses, the rattle of silverware, voices of adults and children who had converged in a common room after a day of play ceased as definitely as if someone had taken the power knob on the radio and turned it off. No one told the kids to be quiet, but they were.

I walked out to find Jeff, but he didn't see me right away. He was making his way around the cement walk that bordered the pool. The cement was completely wet from the afternoon's tidal wave of activity. As he bent to pick up a pair of stray goggles, I could see that the top of his head was sunburned. He got all the way down on his knees and reached into the pool to rescue a floating dragon whose head drooped to one side, and after pulling it to shore, he examined it to determine where the source of its air leak might be. I walked up and stopped next to him.

"Jeff?"

"Hmm?" He continued to palpate the dragon at systematic intervals along its vinyl anatomy. He was probably expecting to hear a question about whether we should have dinner now or later or a request to get more propane for the barbecue.

"Jeff?"

He stood up. His face was flushed from the combination of the exertion of bending and the effects of an afternoon in the sun.

"The hospital just called," I said. Unblinking, he looked at me. "Sarah's had a seizure."

He straightened to his full height then, having been yanked from the satisfaction of completing the small job he'd been doing and transported in warp speed from one reality to another.

I told him what little I knew. He listened. Even in this very personal emergency, Jeff could not shed who he was, a physician as well as a parent. His face didn't wear the panic-stricken look I would imagine another father's might. A man who creates software or stands on an assembly line or practices law would take in this information with an entirely different frame of reference and, most likely, a different reaction. The rational Dr. Blomstedt asked a few questions, but I'd already told him everything I had learned in the three-minute phone conversation. Then his eyes, the father's eyes, looked past me, down to the river, and I could see the light that had sparkled in them all afternoon had disappeared as if my words had blown out the blue-green candles.

I was feeling disoriented and disembodied, almost dizzy. I'd done what I'd intended. I'd delivered the news about our daughter to my husband, but I was waiting to take my next cue from him.

Even in the intensity of the moment, when Jeff started moving again, the pace of his motions was no different from when I'd walked up to him. He placed the dragon in a corner and moved in the purposeful and deliberate way I had seen him do over the years when I had been surprised later to learn that he had been called to some emergency at the hospital.

He put his arm around my shoulders and guided me to the back door of the house. We walked in through the quiet kitchen but didn't stop there. I followed him to our bedroom with feet that felt oddly slow, weighted with each step. In silence we changed from swimsuits and tee shirts to long pants and shirts with sleeves, and I felt silly for ever having presumed to dress for water sports, for a summer day with friends, for tests of manhood.

When I was dressed, I walked back into the solemnity of the kitchen where Kim had resumed feeding the little girls, and the rest looked as if they didn't know what to do. Their shell-shocked eyes stared back at me.

"Can we leave Willie with you?" I asked all of them.

"Of course. Just go. Call us."

Avoiding any hugs that I knew would dissolve the little bit of starch holding me up, I quickly turned and walked out the back door. I was grateful to have these friends at our house, to fill it and keep it warm while we were away. I wondered if I should even tell Willie that Jeff and I were leaving. I thought if he decided to be clingy, I wouldn't be able to bear it, but I had never before left him without saying goodbye. I took a breath and stepped out the back door. I found him playing trucks with Nathaniel, sitting on the grass between the picnic table and the barbecue.

"Bye-bye, Honey," I said. I squatted down to look into his face and ran my hand over the roundness of his head. "Mommy and Daddy are going to the hospital to see Sarah." No reaction. He was making humming engine noises with his mouth and continued to drive his trucks from the sidewalk to the grass, then over the bump from the grass to the sidewalk. "You're going to stay here with Nathaniel and the grown-ups. You'll be having supper pretty soon." He resumed the truck sound effects. I gave him a kiss on his chlorine-scented cheek.

Jeff's goodbye elicited no more emotion from Willie than mine. I walked with Jeff to the garage, and we each opened our doors and sat carefully in our seats. He backed the car out and into the driveway for yet another bleak ride to Springfield.

In the first ten miles of the trip we rehashed what we knew. After that we didn't talk much. Our heads were full of question marks, and there were no answers to be had for the next forty minutes. My silence was a numb freeze, an absence of coherent thought. I simmered with upset and worry as well as anger, though it had no direction. The same words ran like a ticker tape across the inner surface of my forehead: This should not be happening. This should not be happening. She's had no neurological problems whatsoever. Why is this happening?

Jeff drove intently, not speeding, though I wished he would. Most likely he wasn't thinking about driving. I knew he was sorting through the possible causes of the seizure, considering one, ruling out another. We needed more data. He steered with one hand low on the wheel and pushed the turn signal indicator up or down as necessary. He passed other cars and made lane changes with barely a glance in the rearview mirror.

When we got off the highway and stopped at the intersection leading to Baystate, Jeff automatically turned on the right signal. He headed toward the lot we had parked in when we visited Sarah in the winter.

"No, not that way," I said. "She's in the pediatric ICU this time." I told him to turn left into medical center's main parking lot. The ICU for children was different from the ICU for newborns. I had learned when Sarah was in the NICU's intermediate unit that if an infant needed to return to the hospital once it had been discharged, the baby was considered contaminated by the world and therefore disqualified from the NICU. So even though Sarah was as tiny as some of the NICU babies, she could not go back to the neonatal unit. I felt doubly lost, realizing we would have to start all over with nursing staff who were unknown to us and as yet unproven.

After parking the car, Jeff took my hand. We walked into the hospital's main lobby where we stopped at the information desk to ask for directions. The building was new, and we did not know the routine there. We turned and walked as directed like a pair of zombies who'd been programmed to go right, then left, then right again, and I noticed nothing about our surroundings until we came to the elevators. We stepped into the open doors and pressed button number three. We stood in silence while the elevator rose. We stepped out of the elevator on the third floor. Following the signs, we walked down a long, white corridor, and I dreaded what we would come to when we reached its end. We turned the corner and faced a new set of double doors above which the words blared, Pediatric Intensive Care. Without warning, both doors opened, and a young man in blue scrubs walked purposefully through them and past us. He left Jeff and me with nothing but air to push against as we entered the unit.

Intensive care units have a universal technical aura, but each also has its individual feel. The unnatural white of fluorescent light hit first, but there was an ocean-green calm about the individual cubicles. To our right, a man who appeared to be a doctor sat writing at the nursing station desk. I could see from the flecks of gray in his dark hair and beard that he was not one of the young house staff, and when he looked up from the chart that was in front of him and saw us, I could see in his face a careworn, resigned look. We didn't have to introduce ourselves. He nodded once as if to say, "I know who you are."

"She's in there," he said, indicating with his chin which way we should turn, and I heard sadness in those few words.

Sarah had been placed in an isolation room, separate from the other patients if there were any. The unit seemed very quiet, and I noticed that only one other bed was occupied with what looked like a teen-age-sized body that lay in a hump. I could see only lab coats through the glass that divided what must be Sarah's room from the rest of the unit. It looked like all activity on that evening was concentrated in one place. We didn't have to scrub or put on gowns to get into the pediatric ICU, but Jeff and

I stopped when we came to the doorway of the glassed-in cubicle. Except for the beeping of the heart monitor, silence had fallen over the room. In a moment eerily similar to the morning after Sarah's birth when I'd seen her for the first time, the doctors stepped back and a space opened up for us.

When I saw her in the crib, I could not believe it was the same baby I had held and played with the day before. Her eyes were closed, and she lay on her back, completely still. If I hadn't seen the squiggles on the screen and heard the beeping of the cardiac monitor, I would have thought that this pathetic baby had expired, unnoticed, while the doctors stood talking over her body. Her face, neck, arms, and legs were distorted and puffy. Her belly was swollen. She was unrecognizable as our Sarah.

Seeing her naked and exposed, an endotracheal tube coming from her mouth and taped to her cheeks, made me wonder, have I been dreaming since April? I didn't feel as if I were dreaming while I stood there in the intensive care unit, because the moment was all too real and the condition of this baby so closely resembled the one we'd seen much of the previous winter. This seemed to be the true Sarah. Two pads stuck to her chest and one to her abdomen. A tangle of wires led from them to the heart monitor. A steady heart rhythm played across the screen, but the rate was wrong. Like a metronome set too fast, the speed made me uncomfortable. Her chest rose and fell automatically but only with prompting from the ventilator. She took no breaths on her own. A new IV line was taped to one arm. How did they get that in? I wondered. They must have needed another access to her veins when she was in trouble with the seizure. What with emergency medications to stop the seizure, her amphotericin, and IV fluids, the one central line wasn't enough. That alone was disheartening. Clear IV tubing also stuck out from a bulky new dressing that protruded from behind her right ear. Her limbs lay motionless on the mattress in that unnatural, paralyzed-baby position. She was once again held together with tubing and white surgical tape. This did not seem like a dream. What seemed unfamiliar and unreal was the baby of the summer months, the one who had smiled at her brother, slept peacefully through the night in her cradle, and woke happy to spend a few minutes finding her toes with curious fingers.

Like the Saran Wrap that had struck me as odd when I saw Sarah on the morning after her birth, what grabbed me on that August evening was the nontechnical. She lay on the mattress of a large crib, and the side rails of the crib were down. I said the words to myself as if to make sure they were true: a baby in a crib with the side rails down. Nothing held her in a safe place on the mattress as I remembered my mother doing with one hand when she guarded my baby sister, as I would do when Willie and then Sarah lay on the changing table after a bath. There in the pediatric intensive care unit, surrounded by thousands of dollars' worth of lifesaving equipment, the side rails of the crib were in a position that seemed to say there was no threat that she would move, which I interpreted as there is no hope that she will move.

Through the fog that seemed to surround me, I heard one of the doctors say, "We gave Sarah Dilantin to stop the seizure and Valium so we could intubate her. As soon as it wears off, she'll wake up. We can take her off the vent when she starts to breathe on her own." No matter how confident the words coming out of the doctor's mouth sounded, the position of the side rails very clearly told me no one expected this baby to move any time soon.

I reached up to touch her hand, and it was cold. There was no response in her fingers. The hard numbness I had been feeling for just over an hour was shocked alive by the cold of her flesh, and I began to cry. Jeff wrapped his arm around my shoulders, trying to comfort me while he, too, mourned. Looking at the unmoving body, we stood together as if we were at a wake.

After giving his silent fatherly attention to Sarah, Jeff looked up, turned to the physicians who stood in the room, and became a doctor.

"So, what happened?" he asked the room. His voice was calm, but I felt something like a force field surrounding him. What was that energy? Fear? Anger? I couldn't think clearly, and I had to rely on him for that. I wanted to know what he was thinking, now that he'd seen Sarah.

One of the doctors started talking. Sarah's urine output had diminished during her week in the hospital. It had been difficult to monitor the weight of her diapers accurately because she had been having frequent, loose stools after starting the medicines and there had been no way to measure her urine output. Sarah had apparently been retaining fluid over the week and probably not making adequate amounts of urine. It was obvious now that the fungus had been growing for a long time. Most likely the whole process of fluid retention had been simmering long before her hospitalization as well. I thought of Jeff's "fat girl" comment on the Fourth of July. It was just before that weekend that she had developed the sweaty, pudgy look. From the time that her kidney infection had been diagnosed, her weight had increased insidiously from retained fluid and deteriorating kidney function. The human body's normal sodium level is 135-145 mmol / liter. Although Sarah's sodium level had remained relatively stable all summer, for some reason it had dropped precipitously to 115 mmol / liter. Extra water had diluted her blood, and low sodium had caused the seizure.

The small room was crowded with people. There was so much brain power in the cubicle that on one level I felt a strange calm. They had to be able to figure this out. Two of the doctors were nephrologists. They were Jeff's colleagues, and they were fathers as well. They couldn't conceal their own discomfort. The doctor from the desk had also joined the group, and he introduced himself as the unit director. Dr. Stechenberg, the doctor who gave me the results after Sarah's kidney ultrasound, was in the room. She and a resident, perhaps the person who had called me, talked to one another in low tones.

I don't know who led the discussion because my eyes remained fixed on Sarah. I watched her eyelids for any flutter or movement, but there was no sign of waking. Willing those eyes to open, I let my gaze travel from her face down to her toes and back up to her face again.

In order to stop the seizure, they'd given her a number of medications, one of the doctors repeated, and that was why she was asleep and intubated. The doctors assured us again that as soon as the meds wore off Sarah would breathe on her own and the endotracheal tube could be removed.

The murmured speculations continued, and the professional voices drifted to the background. Sarah lay naked on the mattress. Her skin was a blue kind of pale, and her body felt cold and hard to my touch. The side rails of the crib were down. Everything was wrong.

While the doctors scratched their heads and discussed possibilities, a nurse continued to work around the crib, setting up the room for her patient and wiring the unconscious baby to drips and alarms.

"She is a terrific nurse," one of the doctors said to me in a whisper. "So smart. You're lucky to get her tonight. She really should go to medical school." I supposed she was trying to make me feel better, but even in my distracted and unhappy state of mind, those words tweaked the nurse in me. It always rankled when people said that smart nurses should be doctors as if nurses would choose to be doctors if they were intelligent enough, as if being a smart and competent nurse were less important than being a physician. The nurse who circulated around Sarah's crib was obviously skillful. She exuded professionalism and proficiency as she explained in a few words what she was doing to monitor Sarah. She moved with economy, organizing the room and the equipment for her critical patient. There were at least six doctors in the room. They stood talking while one nurse set alarms, checked IV fluids, and measured blood pressure. It didn't look as if Sarah needed another doctor. She needed the best nurse they had to take care of her. I was glad this young woman had not chosen to attend medical school.

One place on Sarah's body not invaded by wires or tubing was her bladder, but that didn't last long. At seven o'clock the nurses changed shifts, and the evening nurse took report and then introduced herself to me. After assessing the baby's condition, she said she would be catheterizing Sarah so her urine output could be monitored. I continued to hold Sarah's cold fingers as the nurse arranged a sterile cloth on a metal tray that stood beside the crib. She grasped the ends of a long package that had been sitting on the mattress and pulled the two ends apart, turning the package upside down. A small urinary catheter dropped onto the sterile towel. After slipping on a pair of gloves, the nurse washed the Sarah's diaper area with a cleansing solution and then changed into a new pair of sterile gloves. She picked up the rubber catheter and dipped the tip into colorless sterile lubricant. With sure hands she inserted the catheter. I winced, but Sarah showed no reaction whatsoever.

The nurse looked at the end of the tubing that she held over a calibrated plastic cup, waiting for urine to drip out.

Nothing happened.

"Huh." She sounded puzzled. She pulled the catheter out and then called over her shoulder, "Can someone bring me a new catheter?" It appeared almost immediately. She opened the new package, dumped the catheter onto the sterile towel, dipped the tip in the lubricant, and inserted it as she had done before.

Nothing again. No urine came from the tube.

Catheterizing a female, especially such a diminutive one, can be tricky, but with a baby who was as cooperative as the unmoving Sarah was, it shouldn't have been too difficult. So the nurse left the second catheter in place, opened a package with yet another catheter and repeated the procedure. Then she knew that one of the catheters was in the right place. One had to be in the bladder and one had to be in the vagina. She again held the end of the catheters over the plastic container, expecting yellow drops. No drops came. She pressed gently with her fingers on Sarah's abdomen, concentrating on the area over the bladder. Nothing came out of the end of the tube. By this time one of the doctors had joined us at the bedside and also looked at the end of the tube. The doctor and the nurse didn't look at each other, and no one looked at me.

The shoemaker's children have holes in their shoes.

That line was back, stalking me, haunting me.

How could Jeff's baby not make urine? Of all the systems to break down—heart, liver, intestines, bones, muscles, blood—how ironic it was that the daughter of the kidney doctor was not making urine.

We knew the specialists who had joined us in the pediatric intensive care unit that evening because they were the same as those who had cared for Sarah in the NICU. At least we didn't have to start all over with them, and they could summarize Sarah's history for the new doctors who would be assuming her care. Through the glass window I could see a resident, or perhaps he was a medical student, sitting at the nurses' station desk. He would occasionally rake his fingers through unruly hair as he pored over a three-inch-thick chart I knew had to be Sarah's.

The evening waned as the doctors came and went from the room. Conversation remained quiet as if the doctors and nurses feared waking the baby from a nap or frightening us with their speculations. Abnormal test results, some too high, some too low, were mixed in with the jargon that floated in the funereal hush of the room: blood pressure elevated; no further seizure activity; no spontaneous breaths; serum electrolytes out of whack; BUN and creatinine, the indicators of kidney function, significantly elevated; no signs of waking. But most puzzling was the lack of urine. She was producing no urine at all.

By eleven o'clock, Sarah showed no sign of waking, but her vital signs had stabilized. The team of doctors had dispersed, and after the flurry of early evening activities, the plan was simply to support Sarah through the night. Tests and procedures were scheduled for the following morning. Jeff said he wanted to go home. His face was drawn, and his tan seemed artificial in the greenish light of the room.

It was too hard for Jeff to stand around in a hospital room and do nothing. In his job, he was one of the team members, one of the doctors responsible for solving problems. He was used to fixing things. After examining a hospitalized patient and writing the day's orders, he moved on to other patients in other rooms. In the office he talked to patients and their families; he gave instructions to nurses; he gathered lab data and test results. He would see fifteen or twenty kidney patients in a typical office day and try to solve their problems. Sitting and waiting in a hospital room was unnatural for him. I told Jeff it was fine with me if he left. Only one of us needed to be with Sarah, and I wanted him to be clear-minded in the morning. So Jeff went home to gather his thoughts and talk things over with our friends. He would have plenty of company there.

At around one in the morning, I lay down on a cot the staff had set up in Sarah's cubicle. The nurses had not asked me if I wanted to stay. They had just assumed I would. I appreciated their unspoken understanding and the small comforts they arranged.

I knew there would be little sleep for me that night, but my eyes were dry and swollen from crying, and it felt good to close them. I pulled the waffle blanket up over my shoulders and rested my head on the hospital pillow that crackled under its cotton pillowcase. My thoughts drifted as the minutes passed, but whenever a new sound broke into my consciousness, my eyes popped open. Eventually I became used to the movements of the nurse, who softened the lights for the night. My final thoughts for the day included gratitude for the attention that had been given to Sarah that night. Intensive care at its best.

Around three o'clock, something unfamiliar agitated the air currents in the room. At first I didn't bother to open my eyes and just listened, but then curiosity forced my eyes open. I was surprised to see the back side of a person in a white lab coat hovering around the crib. He or she, I couldn't tell which, was bent at the waist, apparently working over Sarah.

When I was about to speak, the body moved to the other side of the crib, and I could see that it was a she. She needs to wash her hair, I thought. The young woman's dark hair was pulled back in a skinny ponytail, but she was apparently oblivious to the strands that had escaped to hang limply around her face because she did nothing to tuck them away.

"Hello?" I finally said, which was shorthand for, "Who are you and why are you touching my baby?"

Her head snapped up. I had obviously startled her. I wondered if she had even noticed I was in the room.

"Oh. Um. Hello," she said, finally focusing eyes that hid behind a pair of oversized glasses. She didn't say anything else.

"Who are you?" I had to ask the question out loud since the young woman had not introduced herself or explained her presence.

"I'm the resident on call tonight." I had not seen her with the group earlier. Interns did not rotate to intensive care in their first year in the hospital, but residents did, and the pediatric ICU was on their rotation schedule. I calculated that this young woman had been a resident for six weeks at most, and she looked as if there had been a fair number of nights when she hadn't slept.

Since she didn't volunteer more, I had to ask, "What are you doing?"

"I have to get a blood gas." She hunched forward over Sarah again, but I was low in the cot and on the other side of the crib so I couldn't see what she was doing with her hands. The glasses slipped down the bridge of her nose, and she pushed them back as she leaned forward. In the low, greenish light she looked exhausted and scared. I continued to lie still, but my pulse increased as I watched the resident's uncertainty. She straightened. Hoping she had given up, I held my breath. She walked back to my side of the crib and bent over Sarah again.

Swell, I thought, feeling dismissive of the young doctor and anxious at the same time. Here we are smack in the middle of August, the worst time to get sick. The interns and residents are new, and this one is hovering over my child. I wondered if I would be able to keep my mouth shut. In teaching hospitals, the highest death rates for the year are in July and August when the house staff are inexperienced. Of course she wasn't going to cause Sarah's demise by drawing blood, but I was not feeling kind, and I definitely was not feeling generous enough to offer my baby for an unsupervised teaching experience. Though the resident's skills were as yet unproven, I couldn't help but pull out the mental book I had put on the shelf three months earlier. I gave the evening and night nurses an *A*, but this resident received a *D* for not introducing herself, for her scared-rabbit body language, and, because I was tired, for her greasy hair.

Sarah was in trouble that night—she'd had a seizure and wasn't breathing. She was not making urine. Her problems were magnified by the difficulty of getting to her veins and arteries. Because she couldn't take food or fluids by mouth, her survival depended on getting life-saving measures in through her circulatory system. She needed intravenous access to get medicines in, and she needed intravenous access to get blood out so the doctors had enough information to develop the right care plan. None of the data was stagnant, either. Her condition could change within minutes. Twenty-four hours earlier, when the central IV line had at last been surgically placed, no one had anticipated how important that access would be. The central line helped with getting critical therapies in, but blood can't be removed through the central line. Sarah's superficial veins had been used up and left her caregivers with no good way to get blood samples out.

In an ICU patient, doctors will often sew a special catheter into a wrist artery to deal with just this problem. That catheter, called an arterial line, can be used to draw blood. Once the line is in place, a nurse can connect a syringe to the line and withdraw blood repeatedly without causing any pain to the patient. As a bonus, if a transducer is attached to the catheter, a visual monitor can display information about heart function and blood pressure. In spite of all of the problems she'd had at birth, Sarah had managed to survive her January-through-April hospitalization without an arterial line. They had avoided using an arterial line in the NICU because the down side to such a line was that in a wrist as small as Sarah's, the catheter could interfere with blood circulation to her hand and might leave it permanently damaged. When the doctors were talking over plans for Sarah on the evening of her seizure, Jeff had requested that, if it wouldn't compromise her condition, they try to get through the night without an arterial line. I was surprised. I couldn't bear the blood-drawing torture, and I thought the line was a good idea. But Jeff reminded me that an arterial line could cause her to lose the function of her hand. If she lives, I thought. She isn't even old enough for us to know whether she is right- or left-handed. If Sarah's condition improved by the morning and she started breathing on her own, and if she came off the ventilator as the doctors thought she should, then the arterial line would be unnecessary. Jeff asked if we could revisit the idea of an arterial line in the morning, and the doctors agreed there was no harm in waiting.

I knew why the resident was trying to get a blood sample in the middle of the night. The doctors were trying to wean Sarah from the breathing machine and needed to know if she was getting adequate ventilation. While Sarah was on the ventilator, they would periodically need blood samples to monitor oxygen and carbon dioxide levels. The unfortunate resident had to wrestle with the blood-drawing problem, and the source of her anxiety was obvious. Under the best conditions, getting an arterial sample is even trickier than drawing blood from a vein, and Sarah's condition was seriously compromised.

Trying to detect a pulse in Sarah's wrist, the resident moved her fingers over the skin, stopping in one spot, waiting, moving her fingers a little to the right, a little to the left. Can't she find the pulse? Does that mean she is inexperienced or Sarah's pulse is weak? There were too many unanswerable questions, too many things to be afraid of.

First, do no harm, I thought, willing the young doctor to get the needle in the right place the first time. I knew I would not be able to sit quietly if she was not successful on her first attempt. Wide awake now, I was determined to protect my baby from honest intentions but limited abilities, and I watched every movement the resident made. It had been ten minutes since she'd entered the room, and she continued to move her fingers over Sarah's still wrists and behind her ankles, searching for a pulse she could trust. It was obvious to me she was not confident in what she was feeling in the tips of her fingers. I decided if she picked up a needle and syringe, I would say whatever I had to say to prevent her from doing anything to Sarah without supervision. Then, before I said a word, the resident abruptly turned and left the room. I fell back and closed my eyes. I felt guilty and relieved and then deflated when I remembered that Sarah still needed to have her blood drawn, if not by this doctor then by another.

I pushed aside my blanket, rose from the cot, and walked over to Sarah's bed. My own fingers went to Sarah's cool wrists—first one and then the other—and found the thready, rapid pulse. Staring at this unmoving mannequin of a baby, I stood there for a bit. Then I returned to my cot, lay down, and closed my eyes.

I didn't open them until I heard whispers in the room. From under half-open lids I saw that the young doctor had returned. With her was a man in blue scrubs who, I supposed, was probably her superior. He moved with an air of authority, and I breathed easier with him there. I heard him murmuring to the resident in a quiet baritone as he bent over the crib, and before I could work myself up to being anxious about the painful procedure, the two doctors walked out. One was carrying a syringe full of bright red blood. My relief that the blood drawing was over was immediately overwhelmed by another observation. During what I knew to be a very painful procedure, Sarah had not moved a muscle.

The hands of the clock seemed unwilling to move. If I did settle down in the cot for a few minutes, the piercing of an alarm would jolt me into the present where I was acutely aware of the steady, too-fast beeping that represented Sarah's heartbeat. The alarms didn't last long. Often Sarah self-corrected the breathing or heart problem, and the alarm stopped. If not, the nurse was in the room immediately and took care of the IV or the tubing to the ventilator or whatever might be causing the alarm. As I lay there, tired but wakeful, I had the restless, disoriented feeling that goes with trying to sleep in a strange place. I sat up every now and again to look at Sarah, and I was shocked each time at seeing my baby—who had smiled at me only the day before—laid out in a tragic, foreign body, a body that had betrayed her, a body that had fooled me into trusting the warmth of its smooth skin and alert eyes. The night inched along, and I continued to feel vaguely disoriented as if we had taken one giant step backward and landed in January.

The nurse tiptoed through her work. The doctors had ordered that the number of breaths given to Sarah by ventilator be weaned back in hopes that by withdrawing mechanical assistance, Sarah would have to breathe on her own. Nevertheless, she continued to lie motionless, eyes closed, chest rising and falling only at the command of the machine.

Sometime after four o'clock, I knew I would not be able to sleep. I threw back the cotton blanket and left the room for a change of scene. I pushed the button on the pediatric ICU wall and walked through the automatic double doors I had entered ten hours earlier. I hoped I could find a window to see what the sky said about the night. The corridor turned out to be lined with windows, and the sleeping city was on display through the panes.

I leaned my elbows on a windowsill and stared ahead, but my overtired mind was empty of thought and my eyes registered little of the sky or the city below.

I stayed there for some time, feeling numb and curiously distanced from myself and the situation in the intensive care unit. Sarah's condition was, in my book, "horrible but stable" for the night, and all action seemed to be on hold until morning. It was odd to have everything suspended.

A door opened at the far end of the hall, and I glanced up. A man shuffled down the corridor in my direction. He had a full head of unkempt black hair and a dark beard, and he walked with his head down and almost swaying side to side. He reminded me of a buffalo. He carried a brown grocery bag. I know that guy, I realized, and at the same time it occurred to me that he was almost always burdened with a grocery bag in his arms or an overstuffed pack on his back, except maybe when he was performing tests of manhood in the swimming pool.

It was Jim.

Even when life was going well, Jeff's old friend suffered from insomnia. When he was worried or unhappy, Jim didn't sleep much at all, so I suppose on that night he decided, after staying up three-quarters of the night at home with Jeff, that he might as well drive to Springfield and spend the rest of the night in the pediatric ICU with me. I turned from the window and didn't know whether to laugh or cry. He shifted the grocery bag to one arm and pulled me in with the other. With a brown bag of snack foods crackling between us, I allowed myself to be gathered into the warmth of a much-needed bear hug in the middle of that sterile white hallway. We left the lightening sky behind us and walked back into the pediatric ICU, ready to face whatever the new morning would bring.

I didn't ask if it was okay to have a visitor, and the nurse made no comment when Jim entered the pediatric ICU. He left the grocery bag at the nurses' station and followed me into Sarah's cubicle. Looking at Sarah and all the equipment surrounding her, he stood by the crib. "Oh, Susan," he said, shaking his head, his eyes fixed on the baby. He touched her pale hand and held it in his big brown one. We stood there, mostly silent, for the next two hours.

At seven, Jim convinced me I should go home to shower and change. I could come back later with Jeff. A meeting with all the medical team had been arranged for ten that morning, and they would talk about Sarah's case and what the course of action should be. I allowed myself to be guided out of the hospital and into the car.

I arrived home to the crackling of bacon in the fry pan and the smell of freshly brewed coffee. Kim was having breakfast with the little girls in the kitchen, and though it was just after eight o'clock, Eileen was already in the pool with Willie and Nathaniel. A new day at the summer resort was under way.

When I walked into my bedroom, I could hear the shower running in the bathroom. I stepped out of the clothes I'd been wearing all night, and as I wrapped myself in a robe, I could hear a voice. It was Jeff, talking out loud in the shower. Some people sing in the shower, but Jeff occasionally carries on one-sided conversations. He works out the problems of his upcoming day, practices his side of a debate, or, like the clever chess player he is, develops a number of options in anticipation of someone else's move. He sometimes does this aloud while performing his morning ablutions. I don't know if he's even aware he does it.

When he walked out of the bathroom, I walked in.

"How is she?" he asked.

"The same," I answered.

When I finished washing, shampooing, and rinsing away the previous night, I dried off and stepped out of the bathroom fog to find Jeff standing in front of the full-length mirror in our closet, his neck extended and chin pushed forward as he flipped the lengths of a necktie over, around, and under itself. Wearing a tie wasn't necessarily abnormal, although I thought it a little odd he would choose to wear a tie to the hospital that day. Of course he wears ties to work, but I did not think he was intending to go to work. When he dresses for a day in the office, he usually wears khakis, shirtsleeves, and a tie, often a silly one, a conversation-starter for his patients. On that Thursday, though, he'd chosen a conservative necktie and a white shirt. He was wearing a pair of dark dress pants, and I noticed a matching jacket lying neatly on the bed. It struck me as very strange and a little alarming. Jeff rarely wore a suit. When we got married in Yellowstone, he wore a camel blazer, dark pants, and cowboy boots. On this August morning he looked as if he were going to a wedding. Or a funeral.

"Why are you wearing a suit?" I asked.

He glanced at me in the mirror as if I were challenging him to a duel.

"Because I am," he said. I couldn't read the look in his green-blue eyes. He said no more, moving his attention back to the tie.

"Okay," I said, thinking this subject was definitely not a conversation starter. I asked no other questions and proceeded to pull something considerably less formal out of my dresser drawers.

I ate a little breakfast at Jim's insistence and updated everyone on the night. Jeff and I said goodbye to the group again and drove to the hospital.

When we walked into the unit, I could see men and women in white coats like a posse of medical good guys standing in a horseshoe around Sarah's crib. They included the nurse assigned to Sarah for the day, the director of the unit, Dr. Stechenberg for infectious disease, the nephrologist, and a young doctor I took to be the fresh resident of the day. They were engrossed in conversation. Feeling invisible, I stepped up to the crib. I could see no change in Sarah. Breathing only as prompted by the respirator, she remained unconscious and unmoving.

Jeff eased into the formation. At that moment I understood why he had chosen to wear the suit and what he was talking about in the shower. He had some thoughts about what was going on with Sarah, and he wanted to be heard, not just as Sarah's father but as a physician. He could not very well show up in a white coat, but his medical opinion might be taken more seriously if he looked more like a doctor than a dad. Hence, the suit.

The director of the pediatric ICU was pacing the crowded room. He wanted to do something, it seemed, and the thoughtful deliberation of the specialists was perhaps not his style.

"We ought to dialyze her," he said, almost to himself as he walked back and forth, but the others kept talking. They weren't talking about dialysis as an option, and that puzzled me. Sarah was fluid overloaded and not making urine. Dialysis made sense to me, but neither Jeff nor his nephrologist colleague seemed to agree.

I slipped my index finger into the open curve of Sarah's cold palm. "Sodium, potassium, creatinine clearance," meant nothing as I massaged Sarah's still, cold fingers with my warm, summer-brown ones. I could hear and understand the key nouns as the doctors spoke, but I lost the words in between. What I was beginning to grasp was that the nephrologists apparently did not believe Sarah's blood values or clinical course indicated kidney failure. That meant dialysis was not the answer.

Then what? I wondered, looking at Sarah, not at the doctors. What else is there?

"We looked at Sarah's ultrasound this morning," said one of the doctors. "In all the confusion yesterday, we never got to it. Turns out that her kidneys are grossly enlarged." After being on the medications for a week, the fungus that had filled her kidneys was dying as it was supposed to. No one had anticipated that when the fungus was destroyed by the medication, the residue of the fungus would need to go somewhere. Her kidneys had backed up with urine because a mass of the dead sludge had blocked both kidneys' drainage systems. The kidneys had expanded with a mass of the fibrous, gray glob I had seen a little of in her diaper. That thing had come from her kidneys. Though she wasn't making urine, she didn't need dialysis because her kidneys were still capable of filtering wastes and manufacturing urine, but their outlets, the ureters, were obstructed by the gluey, dead fungus. Hence her swollen little body and the seizure that came from the low sodium level in her blood.

How to get the urine out was the question, and the answer had to come soon. Her blocked kidneys would soon be damaged if the urine did not find an outlet.

The doctors tossed ideas around while Sarah lay oblivious to the attention she commanded. Talking to Jeff as a colleague, they included him in the conversation. When there was a momentary lull, he cleared his throat to speak. Over breakfast I had told him and the others at the table about the resident who had made me nervous during the night and the concerns I had about Sarah being cared for by the house staff. Certainly they were supervised by attending physicians, but they would also make choices and perhaps even do procedures on their own.

Jeff told his colleagues what had been weighing on his mind. "I appreciate that the house staff need to learn and that Sarah is a very interesting case," he said. "We don't mean to be unreasonable parents." He stood with his fingers interlaced in front of his belt buckle and looked gravely around the semicircle from one face to another. "But Susan and I feel that this is not a situation for house staff to manage." Teaching hospitals exist to care for patients, of course, but their mission also includes training physicians in every specialty, nurses, respiratory therapists, phlebotomists, X-ray technicians, and social workers. In some clinical situations, a patient's personal physician will defer to the up-to-date medical technology and knowledge offered by the attending doctors employed by the teaching hospital.

Jeff went on. "Sarah has been through too much and is too sick for us to accept any risks at all right now. We don't have room for any mistakes." He looked around the room, meaningfully, I thought. Had there been mistakes the previous week? Was Sarah in this situation because the doctors hadn't monitored Sarah's urine volume? Should they have catheterized her when the diarrhea started in order to keep track of urinary input and output? Should the nurses have pressed the physicians more about the important measurement that was lost to them?

Except for the mechanical sounds of the monitor and ventilator, the room rang with silence. "We would like to ask that the attending physicians take full charge of Sarah's care and that all decisions be made directly through the attending doctors." He emphasized the word "all." There were murmurs of assent from the group. Jeff's approach had been polite but clear. No one seemed to take offense, and no one argued policy. As the general conversation in the room resumed, I saw Jeff's frame relax for the first time since he had put on the suit coat.

The group discussion had brought the doctors to some agreement in their deductions. Sarah's kidneys were enlarged and blocked but probably still functioning. Most likely, the urine just couldn't get out. She wouldn't need dialysis if her kidneys were working. The doctors needed to demonstrate that the kidneys were, indeed, still functioning.

One of the doctors stepped out of the formation and picked up the receiver on the beige telephone that hung on the wall in the room. He punched in a few numbers and started to talk. I stopped paying attention. Within a few minutes, the person who had apparently been at the other end of the telephone line joined the meeting. He wasn't tall but was definitely imposing with a bulldog look about him. Instead of a white coat, this doctor wore green scrubs, and a surgical mask dangled from around his neck.

Without knowing a thing about the man, my spirits rose. The pediatricians and specialists were thinkers. They tossed around their theories, ideas, and then treatment options for their patient, but their talk could only take Sarah so far. It was eleven a.m., and she had been lying in the same condition for fifteen hours. Now it was time to do something, and the guy in the surgical garb looked as if he was the one to make that something happen.

STENTS

Within thirty minutes, the gathering of doctors dissolved. Jeff and I were left alone in the room with Sarah. The doctors briefed the surgeon on Sarah's clinical situation, and once he'd joined the huddle it hadn't taken long for a plan to formulate. He would take her to the operating room as soon as there was an opening in the schedule, hopefully early that afternoon, to try to prove Sarah's kidneys were still making urine. Then he had to find a way to get the urine out.

Jeff and I stood in silence once the room had emptied, but the slight hope the surgeon had left behind made my ears ring and my head throb. I could hear my heartbeat. I looked up at Jeff's face and imagined there was an intelligent, logical process going on behind his eyes. In contrast, shreds of thought connected and then broke apart in my brain. I looked from Jeff to the QRS complexes marching across the heart monitor screen to the digital numbers on the IV pump to the still body that lay supine on a brand new sheepskin on the mattress. Wishing urine would appear, I stood immobilized by the possibilities. Pee. Yellow drops of body waste. In with the good, out with the bad. I thought about how rarely I sleep through the night without waking in the darkest of the dark to the pressure of a full bladder—first annoying, then insistent—forcing me to slip from beneath the warmth of my covers to tiptoe across the soft pile of the bedroom carpet to the hard tiles of the bathroom floor and the chill of a toilet seat.

Living with a nephrologist caused me to consider urine with uncommon respect. I recognized it as a profoundly underappreciated bodily product. On days when I knew Jeff wouldn't be home until late in the evening, I would take Willie in to see his daddy at the dialysis unit. One chair after another was occupied by men and women with gray complexions, patients who no longer sat on or stood in front of their toilets to pee but instead spent four hours three times a week on reclining chairs where they had their blood filtered of toxins that they would have urinated out if they could have. Shockingly bright red tubing snaked from extended arms and wended its way to a machine that squeezed, churned, and filtered the accumulated by-products of normal metabolism. After those visits to the dialysis unit, I stopped resenting the nighttime calls from my bladder. And at that moment in the pediatric ICU with dry Sarah lying in front of me, I resolved never again to complain about changing a wet diaper.

Six hours later, four p.m. The nurse gently put a hand behind Sarah's back and buttocks and turned her onto her side. With a gloved hand, she removed a soaked gauze pad from the right side of Sarah's lower back. Clear drops of pale yellow liquid dripped from a barely visible pinhole in Sarah's skin.

In the operating room, the surgeon had pierced a tiny opening into one side of Sarah's low back over her kidney. Urine that had been under intense pressure immediately pushed its way through the hole. The flow slowed by the time we saw Sarah back in the pediatric ICU, but drips of urine still oozed out of the invisible opening. The nurse showed us the wet dressing with some satisfaction. Jeff looked intently. My eyes filled, and through the blur I watched in fascination, transfixed by the drops that sprang, one by one, to the surface of Sarah's' skin.

Same day, six p.m. "We don't have many choices," the surgeon told Jeff and me after he joined us in the room where he also watched the urine dribbling from Sarah's back. The day had been long, and we were spent. I wasn't sure I could have made an intelligent choice if there had been one, so maybe it was better that we had few options.

"We will probably have to put in nephrostomy tubes," he said.

"What are they?" I asked, looking at him and then at Jeff. I thought I'd worked with all the tubes there were, but apparently there were some I didn't know about. The surgeon explained that percutaneous nephrostomy tubes were small, indwelling tubes that would be surgically placed through Sarah's low back into each kidney. Allowing constant drainage of urine, the tubes would function as conduits from her kidneys. She would not urinate via her bladder. To manage the dripping, she would have to wear a diaper high up around the lower back to absorb the urine.

"Usually," he added, "the tubes stay in place until a child reaches about two years of age. At that point we can do a surgical repair so she can urinate normally through the bladder." He looked apologetic.

Two years of age. Who could even think that far ahead with this baby? It seemed presumptuous—another surgery when she turned two. At least he hadn't said the word "if" when he talked about her reaching two. Perhaps the surgeon thought we would be horrified by the tubes, but I was too low to worry about problems with diaper changing. A diaper around her lower back? So what. Just do it, I thought. Just get her through this crisis. Then we'll worry about what comes next.

There really wasn't any other plan. Sarah would go to surgery that evening. After the surgeon left, the nurse brought us a sheet of paper that said the hospital had our permission to take our child to the operating room, and Jeff took the pen she offered. Each of us signed. Again.

The nurse set about preparing Sarah for surgery even though everything about her seemed ready except for the paperwork. While we waited I noticed that for the first time since her seizure, Sarah was ever so slightly moving her arms and legs. If I watched her chest closely, I could see she was making her own attempts to breathe between the breaths the machine blew into her lungs. I saw some movements under her eyelids, and they opened a bit for brief moments even though her eyes were unfocused, clouded with medication. Finally, she was waking up.

"Hey, Sweetie," I said, rubbing some warmth into one arm, wondering if she could hear me, hoping my voice could penetrate the pain and confusion that must have felt suffocating to her. I couldn't stop thinking of how uncomfortable she must be as she lay on her back in that relentless position, her other arm stiffly extended on an IV board, more tape around the IV that threaded into a vein in her neck, an endotracheal tube in her mouth and throat, heart monitor pads stuck to her chest and belly. She was not the oblivious baby of February, the baby who did not have even the awareness of a newborn infant. I knew how I felt after two days of being in bed with a viral illness, sore and achy in every muscle and joint. And that was without being attached to any equipment. She must have hurt all over.

The nurse came into the room. "It's time to go," she said. As the nurse and an assistant pushed the crib with the Sarah and all of her equipment to the elevator, Jeff and I walked alongside, unwilling to let her go until we had to. Waiting for the elevator doors to open, we stood side by side in the hallway. Then the doors closed, and our daughter's little parade disappeared.

To pass the time or maybe just to hear myself say aloud what was happening, I told Jeff I was going to call Sarah's pediatrician. Jeff nodded. He had fallen into a chair back in Sarah's ICU cubicle, but I couldn't sit still. I didn't want to go far, and I didn't know what to do. Sometimes doctors at the big medical centers are courteous enough to call the hometown doctor when the condition of their mutual patient changes, but sometimes there is no time. Even a perfectly considerate resident or attending physician could not have called Hugh often enough to keep him abreast of the changes in Sarah's situation on that day. I had already phoned him at home earlier that morning to tell him about the seizure. I arbitrarily chose seven as the time when any physician would be awake. He would want to know, I assured myself to justify my intrusion into the privacy of his morning at home. I wanted to talk with him because with Hugh I didn't have to start from the beginning. And, well, just because.

I went to the pay phone on the wall outside of the pediatric ICU. What a tainted instrument this is, I thought, not really wanting to touch the receiver even as I picked it up with one hand. How often did a parent call from this phone with good news? "She woke from her coma!" or "They saved the kidneys!" or "There doesn't appear to be any brain damage after all!" More likely, in the years it sat there, looking innocent, appearing no different from the phones hanging outside of gas stations or in airports, that telephone had transmitted words that were bleak and emotions that were tortured. Words like "He was hit by a car" or "They found her in the water" then fill in the blank with a parent's worst fear.

From that phone I called Hugh with an update a little more optimistic than it had been in the morning when I'd delivered my own dark, frightened words. Hugh listened, murmured good wishes, and said to keep him posted. Then I made another call and reached the answering machine of the therapist I was scheduled to see the next day. I'd finally been brave enough to make an appointment for myself and now had to say to the recorded voice, "Sorry. I have to cancel. I'm in too much of a crisis to come for therapy." How ironic that was. On my walk back to Sarah's room I felt a little better, but when I saw Jeff sitting in exactly the same position, staring as he'd been doing ten minutes earlier, I plunged right back into the pool of worry.

It wasn't much more than an hour later when the crib rolled back through the double doors of the pediatric ICU. Yanked out of our individual reveries we both stood up, and I looked for something new around or about the baby. After a quick scan of the crib and then Sarah, I thought, with a sinking feeling, she looks no different than when she left. I didn't see any new equipment with the crib, and her quiet, closed face had not changed. I held my questions while the nurse relocated Sarah's crib in her room and attached the ET tube to the ventilator and the wires to the cardiac monitor. Jeff and I eased into our places beside the crib while the nurse did her work, and I looked again for something to feel better about. Then the surgeon burst into the room, "all puffed up as if he had just kissed the Pope's ring," as my grandmother would have said.

"How did it go?" we asked.

The surgeon recounted the way the situation had developed in the operating room. He'd decided to try one last option before going with the plan to surgically insert the nephrostomy tubes. After looking at the ultrasound of Sarah's kidneys yet another time, he had decided to experiment with a nonsurgical solution to the problem of the blocked ureters. "There is nothing to lose in trying," he said. It was surprising to me, because when he had discussed options with us, he hadn't mentioned the possibility of nonsurgical treatment. He probably hadn't wanted to give us false hope. In the operating room, the doctor had taken a tube as long and narrow as a piece of spaghetti, called a stent, and inserted it into Sarah's bladder as he would have done with an ordinary urinary catheter. An X-ray procedure called fluoroscopy allowed him to see the bladder and kidneys on a monitor. He was able to visualize the tiny opening of one ureter, the tube that carries urine from the kidney to the bladder. Then, through some blessed combination of skill, patience, and luck, he was able to direct the stent to the opening of the ureter and guide it into the kidney. With a syringe, he pushed a small amount of fluid through the stent and into the kidney. Happily, fluid returned through the stent, just as the doctor hoped it would. The fluid was colored with the amber of urine, and bits of broken-up fungus from the kidneys as well. As he told the story, I visualized that successful moment in the operating room, and I saw everyone break into applause.

The doctor left the first stent in place and then inserted a second stent into the bladder alongside the first. He located the second ureteral opening and threaded stent number two up into the right kidney. Urine and sludge dribbled out of that stent opening as well. All systems were go. Hallelujah.

This intervention opened up a new avenue of possibilities. If Sarah was producing urine and if the urine could travel from her kidneys through the narrow stents and if the glop that filled the kidneys could be broken up and expelled through the stents in little bits and pieces, Sarah would not have to have surgery to create an outlet for her kidneys. The stents would stay in place both as conduits for urine and a means of treatment. Amphotericin could be directly infused into the kidneys through the stents, and urine and sediment could come out the same way. It might take days, but more likely weeks. Still, the stents were a temporary, nonsurgical treatment. Once the kidneys were clear of infection, the stents could be removed, and Sarah would be almost as good as new.

Back in the pediatric ICU where Jeff and I stood talking to the doctor, Sarah lay flat in the crib, eyes closed to the world, hands open, fingers lax. She still looked more mechanical than human, not showing any sign that something remarkable had just happened to her. Then, as the doctor finished his story, I looked around the perimeter of Sarah's bed again and saw something. A calibrated plastic bag hung low on the crib's rail near the floor quite close to my foot. There was a small puddle of liquid in the bag, and I bent down to look more closely at it. I squeezed the bag. The liquid was a pale and cloudy yellow, and in it floated tiny shards of gray-white sediment. My eyes followed the tubing upward from the bag, and I saw a scatter of droplets clinging to the inside of the clear tubing. A few drizzled together and then rolled into the bag as one big drop. Urine. Pee. Body waste. Liquid gold.

We arrived home late Thursday night with good news to share, but the celebration was subdued. Although the evening's success was much appreciated, the previous twenty-four hours had sucked the joy out of the vacationers.

On Friday, our last evening together, Eileen sat down at the picnic table across from me. I faced the kitchen and could see the rest of the group milling around in the glow of the blue-and-yellow lamps that hung along the room's perimeter. The clank of silverware and rush of water running into the sink accompanied the harmony of their conversation. It felt comforting.

Eileen looked at me and said, "Susan, you have to get a grip on things here. You don't know how long this is going to last. There are two things that you have to do." She spoke with charge-nurse authority.

"What?" I asked dutifully.

"You can't do all of this right now." Her arm swept vaguely out over the universe in general. "First, you have to find somebody to clean your house, maybe even to do some cooking. Second, you have to find someone to take care of Willie so you can do what you need to do with Sarah down in Springfield. Maybe you can even get someone to come here to the house to do both things."

Numb at the prospect of having to make something happen, I nodded my head.

"Good idea," I said out loud, but I secretly did not think I really had the energy to make such arrangements. Putting an ad in the newspaper, being home to answer the phone for responses, interviewing a babysitter, checking references. I had trouble considering the possibility of leaving Willie with someone I might find through the newspaper. How many references would be enough? The planning seemed daunting. Emotional strain had drained my strength. I knew my finger couldn't dial the phone, and my mouth wouldn't say the words I needed to say to make any of it happen. I could not think beyond the next morning when our friends would drive out of our driveway. Their spirit kept the house vibrant over the week. I dreaded the thought of how empty the house would feel without them.

The group interrupted my conversation with Eileen when they filtered out to join us at the picnic table. In the glow of the citronella candles the six of us talked until mosquitoes finally won and drove us indoors. Then it was time for packing and bed.

There were no surprises the next morning—breakfast, clean up, and the hustle of getting cars organized. We shared last minute promises to call, keep in touch, send easy recipes. Then, all Jeff, Willie, and I could do was watch the winking of brake lights for the last time as our friends disappeared from our driveway and left us on our own.

SEPSIS

Sarah should have turned the corner after she began producing urine. She should have peed out the extra fluid that caused her arms and legs to swell and her face to become that of a stranger. She should have started breathing on her own and then been extubated, getting rid of that damned tube and the ventilator that went with it once and for all. Then she should have started drinking milk from a bottle and getting some fuel into her system. She should have been alert, looking around the room, fussy to be somewhere else. She should have been sitting on the lawn in our backyard and feeling the tickle of late summer grass behind her knees.

Instead, she got a fever. While Jeff, Willie, and I stood in the driveway hugging our friends, promising to call, thanking them for everything, we were unaware that a new storm was brewing in Sarah's veins. We walked back into a house still reverberating with voices, music, and clanking dishes, and I called the pediatric ICU to see how Sarah was doing.

"She's developed a fever," the nurse at the other end of the phone said. "We're working it up."

Damn. I was hoping Sarah would begin to improve once the urine problem was solved. I was not expecting a fever.

The vacationers had left the place shipshape, so there was no major cleanup for us to do. Jeff went off to throw sheets and towels into the washing machine, and I gathered the paraphernalia Willie would take to Grandma and Grandpa's house, where he would spend the afternoon while Jeff and I went to the hospital. Before long, we were packed up and heading south.

The day looked like the summer version of the one in January when my father had driven me away from Baystate. Gray. It was a dull, gray morning. As we drove south, I caught occasional glimpses of the Connecticut River. The water was gray without a glint of light on its surface. The sky was gray. The air seemed gray with the moisture that hung in it. The leaves on the trees didn't have enough green power to project any color beyond themselves. By the time we reached Enfield, the clouds seemed nearly to touch our heads. The air was so heavy I wished the rain would just let loose and spill to the earth instead of smothering us in a steamy cloud.

Willie was the ever-adaptable child that day. He'd slept for most of the hour-long drive and then allowed himself to be carried into Grandma and Grandpa's house as if this visit were his idea. A sleepy smile played across his round face when he spied his Grandma. Have bubby, will travel, I thought, seeing him clutch the treasured blanket from the comfortable altitude of Jeff's arms. I felt sad at having to leave him since he'd been left behind a lot that week, but he seemed so completely happy as my mother fussed over him that I couldn't even muster any guilt.

Jeff and I were quiet on our way to Springfield. I was bereft. Our son was with his grandparents. Our daughter was in the hospital. Our friends had departed. Having them at our house for the week allowed me a certain distance from the urgency of Sarah's condition. Now I was crashing head-on into reality where there seemed was no end in sight to Sarah's illness.

We were shielded from the weather in the air-conditioned car for the fifteen minutes it took us to drive to Springfield. But when I opened the car door, I felt as if a wall of heat and humidity hit me in the face. There couldn't possibly be enough oxygen in air so saturated with moisture. It was so humid I couldn't take a breath deep enough to satisfy my lungs. Jeff reached for my hand, and we walked toward the hospital. My body felt heavy, and my feet felt slow. I guess I wasn't looking ahead as we walked, because Jeff suddenly stopped while I continued to move forward. I looked up to see why.

"Hey, Patrick!" he said.

Jeff's friend stood directly in front of us on the sidewalk near the hospital's main entrance. A stethoscope hung around his neck, and he looked relaxed, a casual Saturday doctor in shirt sleeves.

"Hi, guys," he answered, but with only a fleeting rendition of his usual twinkle.

"Do you have patients here?" I asked. Usually his patients were admitted to Mercy Hospital, a five-minute drive away.

"Well, sort of," he answered. "I needed to check on an X-ray, but I mostly wanted to see how your little one is doing." He hadn't seen Sarah since he and Deedy babysat for her on the night of Elaine's wedding in June. He looked at each of us. "She's really struggling up there, isn't she." It wasn't a question, and I felt a familiar sinking sensation. There were brief moments when I fantasized Sarah's condition might improve and I would walk in to a happy surprise. An awake baby who was breathing on her own was what I was looking for on that day. But Patrick's face and voice told us we would not be seeing a big turnaround when we walked into the pediatric ICU.

As we stood on the sidewalk, I half heard his conversation with Jeff, but it faded into the background as I thought about how there was something so tender and sweet about a grown man going to visit a baby in the hospital. She wouldn't know him. She wouldn't smile at him. She wasn't even conscious. The kindness made me want to sit on the curb and cry.

My thoughts returned to the conversation, and I listened as Jeff and Patrick talked.

"Well, Deedy was really worried, and she wanted me to come," he was saying. "She knew you had enough on your minds and didn't want to call you. I'm the scout."

We caught up on family news, then hugged our friend and parted. I took a breath and turned toward the hospital entrance with new resolve. Our visit with Patrick may have been short, but it seemed to carry healing powers. A little Band-Aid over a big wound, but it helped hold the raw edges together.

Forty-eight hours after getting her immunizations, Sarah had developed a fever, and it seemed she grew sicker each day after that. I recapped the history in my mind as we walked to the elevator. Immunizations. Fever. Fungus. Hospitalization. Toxic medications. No IV sites. To the operating room for a central line. A seizure. To the pediatric ICU. On the respirator. Blocked ureters. No urine. Now urine but still unconscious. No spontaneous breathing. More fever.

By the time she'd stopped putting out urine it didn't seem possible she could get any worse and still be alive. The pediatric surgeon found a way to treat the urine problem, but now she had developed a fever.

On some level, I had become used to the negatives. Each new problem and its technical or pharmacological solution layered itself insidiously over the previous one. Hearing Patrick say Sarah was struggling allowed me to see her condition through his eyes, and he knew what the names and numbers meant. When I walked into the unit and saw her, I agreed with Patrick. It was hard to imagine Sarah could look worse than she had the day before, but she did.

She was still on the respirator. Her temperature had spiked, and her blood cultures grew out *Klebsiella* and *Citrobacter*, strains of potentially lethal bacteria. They had probably invaded as a result of the manipulation that had gone on during the kidney procedures and because of her general vulnerability. The names of the bacteria didn't mean as much to me as knowing they were colonizing in her bloodstream. It was one thing for her to have an infection localized to the kidneys; it was another to have bacteria in the circulatory system, where they multiplied exponentially. Her white blood cell count had jumped to 42,000 (normal 15,000); her temperature had spiked to 101 degrees (normal 98.6) and then dropped to 96 degrees because her body was too sick to mount the proper reaction to the bacteria. Her blood pressure also hit a new low of 62 / 34 (normal 90 / 60). In order to fight back the infections, two new antibiotics dripped into her IV lines. One I didn't pay attention to, but the other was the gentamicin that she'd received as a newborn. Gentamicin was the antibiotic that could cause hearing loss and kidney failure in infants.

Even with the challenge of infection, the doctors were trying to get Sarah off the respirator, and she was actually showing signs of trying to breathe on her own. She set off the pressure alarms on the ventilator by trying to take breaths in between the ones the machine dictated. But her efforts remained inconsistent, and when the nurse turned down the number of breaths per minute that would be delivered by the machine, Sarah regressed to having spells of apnea and bradycardia.

Jeff and I stood like zombies next to the crib. Time dragged without any discernible improvement in Sarah's condition. She made very little progress with weaning from the machine which still did most of her breathing. At the change of shift, the afternoon nurse, Marianne, came in to check Sarah's vital signs. I liked her. She was lively and very competent around Sarah. Listening for a blood pressure, she bent over Sarah's arm. When I asked what the pressure was, Marianne looked up and said it was barely discernible to her ear or her fingertips.

My stomach had already been queasy. Watching the numbers that were all wrong as they flashed on the monitors, I felt a witch's brew of fear and panic mixing and growing inside of me as I stood next to Sarah's crib. Being stuck there at her bedside was worse than being at a horror movie when I knew the bad part was coming. I wanted to shut my eyes and clap my hands over my ears until whatever was going to happen was over. In contrast to my insistence on being awake for the C-section at Sarah's birth so I could be there no matter what happened, I couldn't do it any more, not on that afternoon. I wanted general anesthesia, to wake up when it was all over, whatever it was, whatever all over might mean. I knew I should stay there with my child, but the room was closing in around me.

"I have to get out of here, Jeff."

He looked down at me. "Do you want to go to the cafeteria for a while? Get a cup of coffee?"

"No. I need to go home. I can't stay any more."

He looked at me and nodded. I looked at Sarah one more time, squeezed her thin arm, and walked out of the room. Jeff lingered a bit, probably to tell Marianne we would be at home if she needed us. He joined me in the hall outside of the unit, and we walked away in silence.

When we stepped out of the climate-controlled medical center, the afternoon was still heavy and gray, worse than it had been earlier if that was possible. The sky seemed to press down on my head. The humid air felt like clammy hands that touched every inch of my skin and caused my shorts and shirt to stick to my body. It took everything I had to walk with any control to the car. I wanted to run from the hospital, from the beeps and mechanical breaths, from the baby, from the air that surrounded me.

We went to retrieve Willie. Mom invited us to stay for supper, but I was obsessed with wanting to be at home. We gathered Willie and his things, got into the car, and turned northward. Route 91 took us past Exit 10, the one that would have taken us back to Baystate if we wanted to go there, and I felt a tug when we drove past it. We can go back for a quick peek at her, I thought. We can take turns, one of us staying with Willie in the waiting room while the other goes up to the unit to check on her just once more. But I didn't say anything as we drove by the exit, and neither did Jeff. The Red Sox announcer droned on the radio for the duration of our sixty minutes in the car, but I could not have reported the score or even the name of the opposing team when the ride was over.

It was after eight o'clock that evening when the phone rang. Jeff and I were still circulating around the kitchen. He was washing pots and pans while I loaded dishes and silverware into the dishwasher. Though my brain told me to respond to the ring, my legs wouldn't carry my body towards the telephone. I didn't want to talk to anybody, and I didn't want any bad news from the hospital. Jeff dried his hands, walked to the phone, and picked up the receiver. I knew from his voice that it was not a social call. I turned, slowly let my body lean back into the kitchen counter, and tried to make sense of his side of the conversation.

"Yes, it is. Oh, yes. Oh. Uh huh." A long silence. Then he asked a few questions, but they were weightless without the words that I couldn't hear from the other end of the line. I waited, not moving.

He said goodbye and placed the receiver back on the wall.

"She's having a little bleeding around her central line tonight," Jeff said. "They're giving her a transfusion of platelets." Platelets are the components that cause blood to form clots.

He didn't say how much or how long she'd been bleeding, and I couldn't bring myself to ask. We finished doing the dishes.

On Sunday morning when Jeff and I went back to the hospital, Marianne was at Sarah's bedside again. She looked at me with eyes that didn't try to hide what she was thinking.

"Well," Marianne said, and with some heat in that one word, I thought. She looked away from me to cancel the alarm that told her the IV medication bag was empty. "I was wondering when you were going to get here." Marianne had worked the evening shift and was back to work days. Jeff had stopped to talk with a physician who sat at the nursing station, so I was on my own with the upset nurse. Wondering what I'd done wrong, I felt acutely uncomfortable.

"What's going on?" I asked, taking hold of Sarah's fingers, which were warm for a change, and checking her out from head to toe. Skin color better. Two IVs dripping. Urine in the bag. Her face. Something about it was different.

Marianne's eyes flashed as she moved around the crib, but she did not look directly at me as she focused on Sarah's equipment. "Well, it was touch-and-go for a while last night, and I kept expecting you to come in."

The phone call. Had Jeff not told me something? But even if he was trying to protect me, wouldn't he have come in himself if the doctor had told him there had been a critical change in Sarah's condition?

I stood rooted to the floor and then found my tongue and said to Marianne, "I didn't know. What do you mean by touch-and-go?" Her eyes looked quizzical then, as if she were trying to figure this out. Bad night for the baby. Parents never even came in. A doctor and a nurse! Where were they? Didn't they get it? Didn't they know? She was probably trying to decide if we were callous, uncaring, or irresponsible.

"What happened?" I asked, fighting the feeling in my stomach even as I observed that Sarah looked better than she had the day before.

The story poured out. Once Marianne started talking, she couldn't stop. She said that late Saturday afternoon, after Jeff and I had gone home, she'd noticed that the dressing covering Sarah's central IV line had become stained with blood. When she changed the dressing, she noticed more blood seeping from the place where Sarah's intravenous line exited her skin. Even when Marianne applied pressure, the bleeding didn't stop. The doctor on call ordered a blood test and found that Sarah's platelet count had dropped precipitously. We knew from the phone call that her platelet count was down, but I didn't know the number. Her blood was not clotting. Marianne said that she had stayed beyond the end of her shift until two in the morning after a long and frightening evening with Sarah.

Marianne seemed to calm down with the recounting of the events of her harrowing shift. While she was speaking about my child, I knew exactly what she was talking about. I pictured my hands, like hers, hanging the bag of platelets for a little boy, adjusting the drip rate, putting pressure over the seeping wound, hoping the bleeding would stop, knowing it hadn't. It was like a silent movie playing in a black-and-white memory, a scene colorless except for the stain of red that kept appearing and growing. I saw my gloved hand remove a bright red gauze pad from the boy's chest. He also bled from the place where his central line was inserted. He was only two and had been in the Yale pediatric ICU for over a week with severe asthma and infection. His lips were blue, and I tried to convince him that he needed to wear the "Halloween mask" that delivered the oxygen he needed.

Marianne's voice came back to me. "We put a pressure dressing over the line," she said again, "but she just kept bleeding." I saw her hand, and mine, remove one soaked square of gauze and replace it with another. I hoped the new one would be the last as I had walked away from the bedside to gather more gauze and tape. When I returned to the boy, a bright red stain was spreading from the center of the white gauze. It began its creep until the red edged out the white. I removed that square of gauze and replaced it with another. And then another. He died that night.

This was a new problem to add to Sarah's list: DIC. Disseminated intravascular coagulation. Sepsis, the overwhelming numbers of bacteria in her bloodstream, had caused her blood to lose its clotting factors, and because the blood refused to coagulate, she was at risk for hemorrhage. She could have bled from a vulnerable place at any time, and if bleeding started, there might not be enough fingers to hold back the flood.

Where the hell were we? I wondered, furious not to have been there, relieved not to have been there, because I couldn't have stood there, watching her bleed. I knew exactly how Marianne felt about us not being there. Did Jeff not tell me enough last night? Did he know the extent of Sarah's condition? Had the resident not told him enough? I had been an ostrich. I hadn't asked any questions. But I had no strength on the previous evening. I had no will. I had no ability to deal with what they might tell us. So, I hadn't asked.

We should have been here, I thought. What if Sarah had died? I wanted to slap myself. And yet I knew that I couldn't have managed anything more. I couldn't have stood there and watched her bleed.

As frightening as Marianne's story was, there was a sense of unreality as I listened to her, because I could see as I stood at Sarah's bedside that her condition had stabilized.

Once she'd told me about Sarah's night, Marianne seemed to forgive Jeff and me for not being there. My shock had to be obvious, and maybe that was enough for her. Marianne settled back into the routine rituals of Sarah's care, and I looked at Sarah more carefully. There was no bleeding from anywhere that I could see. Sarah had a bulky but very white dressing taped over the site of the central line at her neck and shoulder. Her color seemed better than it had the day before. In fact, I felt the first signs of something positive in Sarah's appearance. What was it?

It was her face. I could finally see her face, and when I looked down after Marianne stopped talking, I saw that Sarah's eyes had opened. Her eyes met mine, straight on. No smile yet, but there was something else.

"The endotracheal tube." I looked at Marianne. "It's gone?"

The nurse smiled for the first time.

"It is." She turned to Sarah and began speaking to her in a direct, respectful, talk-to-the-baby voice. "Tell Mummy all about it, Sarah. You tell her. They took out that ugly old tube last night, didn't they?"

Somehow, even with the confusion of the bleeding, transfusions, and lab tests taking place at her bedside on Saturday, Sarah had been weaned from the ventilator late in the evening. I could hear her breaths then, wheezy and musical, as she moved air through an airway swollen after nearly a week of being on the respirator. Sarah stared at Marianne as she spoke. Sarah wasn't quite ready to talk yet, but she was certainly listening.

The combination of plasma and other fluids dripping into her veins had worked. Her clotting factors were approaching normal. She was breathing on her own. The tiny catheters that drained urine from her kidneys were taped to the inside of her thighs and then pinned to the sheet so as not to pull on her. She had to be uncomfortable with a fiery throat, stents in place, and muscles probably stiff and sore from lying in one place on the mattress all week. She did not cry nor did she smile. Breathing once again on her own and looking more serious than any baby should, she lay there in her crib surrounded by IV pumps, monitors, and alarms.

My greatest fear during both hospitalizations was that Sarah would not be able to come off the respirator. What kind of decision would we have to make if she could not be weaned? How much time would have to pass before we would make that decision? If she could breathe on her own, I felt that we could handle almost any other complication. I was, therefore, almost deliriously happy that she had been extubated and I could see her entire face again. Without the tube she looked like herself. Bits of gummy tape residue adhered stubbornly to her cheeks and chin, and I had to fight the urge to search for an acetone pad to rub the sticky stuff off so she didn't look so messy. I didn't want Marianne to think I was being critical of her care, though, so I held myself in check and just talked to Sarah.

She stared back at me. With her eyes open, she looked as if she had moved back inside herself once again. I looked into those grave eyes for the first time since she'd had the seizure and wondered, as I always did, what was going on behind them.

Jeff joined me at the crib side. Sarah shifted her eyes to him without moving her head.

"Hi, Little One," he said softly as he slipped his finger into the crescent of her hand. She stared at him without changing her expression. There weren't many body parts she could move, so she just held on with one little fist and her eyes while her breaths whistled through her swollen trachea.

I stood back a little, thinking about infant bonding as I had done many times in the previous nine months. Much has been written about the connection that forms between infants and their mothers from the moment of birth. I believed all of it when I had been a young nurse preparing women for their birth experiences and then when I became a mother to Willie. Jeff had held Willie immediately after he was delivered, and I had nursed him for six months before he ate a bite of solid food. We had bonded, I thought, according to the books. So what about Sarah? Where did that leave us and her? Would we have the connection we needed? Sarah had not been held at all for the first month of her life, and when Jeff and I did finally get her out of the isolette and into our arms, it had been a major ordeal. Being held was another procedure she'd had to endure, more like a trip to the X-ray department than a soothing cuddle. Not only that, but how could she interpret all of the pain, the lights, the noise that she had experienced in the past two weeks, and in much of her first year, as anything but torture? Why should Sarah consider her life experience differently than an abused baby might? And now, being hospitalized after having lived in the sweet haze of a life at home where we snuggled and serenaded her, how could this isolation from her family make her feel anything but abandoned and hurt?

I didn't know the answers to those questions. There were so few babies of Sarah's birth weight who had survived that I doubted researchers had a sample of children large enough to study. Standing there at her bedside, I had to shrug off those worries. It didn't matter. We would hold her again and love her. We would let her know where she fit in our family and in the bigger world around her. We would feed her, keep her warm and safe, and protect her in any way we could. Jeff and I were well aware of how little control we had over her life or over any of our lives, and how many things for which there was no protection, but we would do everything we could. From the unflinching look in Sarah's eyes as she looked at her father on that Sunday morning in August, it seemed obvious that he and his child had some kind of connection. I had to believe that, in Sarah's case, we would prove the experts were just plain wrong.

AUTUMN

When Sarah experienced the seizure and all of the events that followed, it was as if Jeff and I had plunged into the ocean with stones in our pockets and sunk down into churning water. On the weekend when Sarah had become septic and her blood pressure had dropped, her blood would not coagulate, and it seemed that life was seeping from her body. She hit absolute bottom. There were no other options, nowhere else for her to go. Jeff and I held her hands and descended with her.

We didn't know Sarah had gone down as far as she would go on the night of her infection and the clotting problems, the night life threatened to leak out of her veins drop by drop. On the Sunday when, dejected and hopeless, we'd dragged ourselves into the hospital, we found with considerable surprise and some disbelief that the direction of Sarah's trajectory had changed. The antibiotics had started to work, her blood had regained its ability to clot, her temperature had come closer to normal, and her kidneys were once again producing good urine. Perhaps the shoemaker's child would find her shoes after all.

Sarah spent twenty-nine days in pediatric intensive care. Once the calendar turned to September, she improved steadily each day. Her color came back from the sallow shade of illness. Her eyes brightened and focused on her surroundings and the people in her life. Once she began to show some interest in what was happening around her, we decorated her crib with stuffed animals and a mobile and the plastic bird that played tinny songs when visitors pulled his string. Her day was busy with nurse-directed activities that included vital signs, weight checks, and frequent adjusting of the stents; daily visits from pediatric residents, infectious disease doctors, and kidney doctors; and trips to the radiology department where specialists bent their heads over her X-rays and dye studies. Progress in her kidneys was measured by their decreasing size and the millimeters of receding sludge. Respiratory therapists, social workers, and God only knew who else brought their special skills to her. She took medicines by mouth and intravenously every day.

What kept Sarah in the intensive care unit were the stents that threaded up into her kidneys. She was not in any acute danger once she was extubated and the bleeding was controlled, but she was still getting IV antibiotics and the stents were a hassle to work with. They alone required too much nursing care to be manageable on the general pediatrics floor. The pediatric ICU nurses had to fiddle constantly with the drainage, which was often clogged by the fungal debris still getting sloughed out from her kidneys. Each catheter was attached to its own drainage bag so the nurses could see if one tube or the other had stopped draining. If the tube going into the right kidney plugged, the nurse would fill a large syringe with a measured amount of sterile water and flush the tubing till the plug moved and the tube drained. Then, more than likely, the nurse would notice that the left tube had plugged up again because of the constant breakdown of sludge. The process would have to be repeated on that side. And so the day went. But Sarah's temperature had normalized, and her blood pressure was stable. Her lab results showed significant improvement in kidney function. She was stuck in intensive care not because she was acutely ill any more, but because of the one-on-one attention her equipment demanded.

I traveled to Springfield whenever I could. Willie went to Lynda's every morning, and on days when she had an extra opening, he would stay through the afternoon. Either Jeff or I would go back to the hospital in the evening. Unlike Sarah's first months in the hospital, it now felt as if she really knew when we were there and very likely knew when we were absent, as well. When either of us walked into the room, she greeted us with smiles of recognition.

In spite of all of the activity that surrounded her, she napped on and off during the day. The nurses told me that she slept well after they softened the lights at night. One day, all of a sudden, her appetite returned. Then I held her whenever I could and offered her a bottle when the nurses said it was time. She sucked down formula with enthusiasm. When awake, she sat in her infant seat, paying attention to her small world. Sometimes she played with a toy that Marianne had given to her, a "diamond ring." It was a squishy mini beach ball of red, blue, and yellow about three inches in diameter with a foam center and attached to a fabric-covered foam ring that could slip onto Sarah's wrist or ankle. Marianne hoped if Sarah had a bright bauble on her wrist, she might be tempted to lift and wiggle her hand and arm to get a view of the entertainment strapped there. Before Sarah had become sick, she had been reaching for toys and toes, and Sarah's ever-vigilant nurse hoped to stimulate that kind of play. As Marianne straightened bed sheets, measured fluids, and adjusted equipment around Sarah's crib, I heard her tell her tiny patient, "When you grow up, Little Girl, you should expect to see a diamond no less than the size of that beach ball on your finger."

Then she'd take Sarah's wrist and wave it in the air so the bell inside the beach ball would jingle and dance.

We started to hear Sarah making conversational, even happy, sounds. The doctors, consultants, and nurses who had been a part of her history came by to visit, and she sized them up and then surprised them with eyes that crinkled and a toothless smile. One day I walked in to see the housekeeper, a short, round, and usually tired-looking woman, leaning over the crib and having an animated chat with Sarah.

Although all appeared to be going better, I still walked around with my fingers crossed. I was unable to let myself totally relax into the belief that her recovery would continue smoothly. My fears seemed justified one morning when Dr. Stechenberg joined me at Sarah's crib. Getting right to the point, the doctor said the left kidney appeared clear on ultrasound imaging but the right contained white material they could see better now that swelling in the kidney had decreased. The doctors were concerned that the white stuff could possibly be new fungal formations. My anxiety meter spiked automatically, but in the weeks since Sarah's low point in August, she had made such steady progress that I couldn't work up the energy to go into a full-blown panic. Dr. Stechenberg downplayed the imaging findings, and I felt as if even she was unwilling to believe it could all happen again.

The doctors regularly repeated the urine cultures and kidney tests. Eventually the nephrologists, intensive care doctors, radiologists, and infectious disease people put their heads together, checked the findings, and concluded the white tissue was more likely to be scar tissue than new fungus. Sarah's lab values showed that her kidney function was getting close to normal, and on September 9, a nephrostogram—an X-ray that pushed dye into her kidneys to check the placement of the stents— showed that all of the fungal sludge was gone. What had been a grossly swollen drainage system had finally decompressed, and although Sarah's kidneys were still somewhat enlarged, they were on their way back to normal function.

At the end of the second week of September, the doctors discontinued the stents. The tiny catheters were pulled from her kidneys, and Sarah was transformed once again into a baby who needed to have her diaper changed instead of having her catheters flushed every few hours. She was nine months old, and, having lost all of the excess fluid she'd been holding over the summer, she weighed barely eight pounds.

She still had to complete a full ten-week course of IV therapy with amphotericin b to eradicate any fungal spores that might hide in the recesses of her kidneys. By the time her stents were pulled, she'd received almost six weeks of the medication. Since her equipment was now down to just IV lines and an apnea monitor, the doctors said she could be moved out of the intensive care unit to the pediatrics floor.

As worrisome as it had been to have her in intensive care, I'd felt secure in the constant presence of the staff in that setting. My feelings about Sarah being moved to the general pediatrics floor were confused with memories of Sarah's discharge from the NICU in April and her move to the Franklin Medical Center in May. Even though those experiences had gone well, I couldn't get past my anxiety over the inevitable move from the pediatric ICU. The general pediatrics floor was very busy. There were questions that still lingered like an itch I could never quite reach, and I felt I needed to be there to watch Sarah as well. Had Sarah been observed closely enough the week she was on the floor? Had the nurses noticed her weight gain? Had they reported the frequency of her diarrhea and the inability to measure her urine output? And if the nurses did report and record all of that, had the doctors paid attention? Could anything have been done to avoid the chain of events that sent Sarah to the ICU?

I would have preferred to stay with Sarah all day, but with Willie at home, that was not an option. In addition to my worry about Sarah getting less attention on the pediatrics floor, I did not want to continue a schizophrenic life, mothering Willie at home and then traveling to Baystate until Sarah's medical treatment was complete. Though I should have been grateful just to have her alive, I didn't like the thought of this hospital routine continuing for another month.

Then one day, a bulb flickered in my head, like the ancient, round fluorescent one on my grandmother's ceiling. It would sputter with flashes of light for the first few seconds after I flipped the wall switch to on, and I watched the white circle with a child's anxiety, not convinced it really would come on.

Hey, Susan, I reasoned, you are a nurse. I had to remind myself that not only was I a nurse, but I'd even been a nurse in pediatric intensive care. The bulb brightened. You are as qualified as anyone on the pediatrics floor to take care of your baby. Once Sarah was out of the intensive care unit, she would have no special equipment but the central venous catheter and the apnea monitor, and I was comfortable with both of those. She would need to have the medicine infused each day. There was nothing magic about the hospital. I knew that at home I could provide her with the care she would need, and all of us would be much happier.

I could hardly wait to talk to Jeff the day of my revelation. "Do you think they would let us bring her home to do her treatments?" I asked him. "We could even take her to Franklin each day for her IV therapy if we have to."

He shrugged his shoulders. "I don't think it would be a problem to do her treatments at home," he said. So the next day, when Dr. Stechenberg came to see Sarah on her morning rounds, I repeated my question to her.

"What do you think about Sarah having her IV therapy at home?"

I was relieved to see that she did not look shocked, and she did not need to mull for very long over my proposal.

"Let me make a few phone calls," she said. She gave Sarah's bootie a little squeeze and swept out of the room.

It went just as I had hoped. In fact, the whole process unfolded so quickly I could hardly believe it was happening. A social worker met with me to talk about Sarah's discharge needs and arranged a time for me to meet in Sarah's room at Baystate with the pump nurse, who would teach me how to use a portable IV pump. In less than twenty-four hours, the nurse who specialized in equipment and procedures for outpatients was teaching me how to mix the medicine and place it in the pump. Just two days after I had made the proposition to Dr. Stechenberg, I was standing at Sarah's bedside, preparing to assist the floor nurse as she changed the sterile dressing over Sarah's central line.

Sarah would be discharged on Monday, September 15. With my head buzzing a little, I drove home from the hospital on the afternoon of the dressing demonstration. I had the feeling that my hands were not really controlling the steering wheel, my foot not really touching the gas pedal. Sarah's place on the planet seemed to be all turned around. Her life in the hospital was real. Her anticipated life at home was fantasy, like going to Disney World. The ride home passed in an eye blink. If the trip had been as quick each day I'd visited her in Springfield, the distance wouldn't have seemed such a burden. I turned off the highway at Exit 27, drove the roads of Gill that took me to Lynda's house, retrieved Willie, and arrived home all in a pleasant fog.

As I prepared Willie for bed on the evening before his sister was due to leave the hospital, I told him the story of how Sarah would come home the next day to be with us and how Mommy would not have to be gone so much anymore. Continuing my chatter in an attempt to distract him, I pulled his tee shirt over his head before he could protest. The shirt was off in a flash. Looking into his round face to determine what registered in his two-year-old mind, I saw not questions or interest but eyes too bright. I touched his forehead, his cheeks, his chest, but I didn't need to. I didn't need a thermometer, either. His body had that familiar, too-warm glow.

The ramifications of this fever hit me at once, and my heart sank with a thud. As I looked at Willie's flushed face, I saw myself hiding in the attic with Sarah in May in an earlier version of this circumstance. What a neurotic, crazed woman I'd been then, and I didn't want to do that again. I was so looking forward to Sarah's homecoming, but her return would just have to be put on hold. I knew that, as disappointing as it might be, I could survive if she had to stay in Springfield for a few more days if that was safer for her.

I took Willie into the bathroom and wet a washcloth. He tolerated a few swipes across his face but drew in his breath when I swabbed his chest, belly, and his back. I tried to be quick. The cloth was warm, but his body was warmer. I looked at him closely. No rash. No runny nose. No cough. I slipped a thermometer under his arm for a few minutes and distracted him with more talk. Then I took a look at the mercury, trying to get it in a position where it wasn't blurry. One hundred and one degrees. That would equal about one hundred three rectally. Hmm. I didn't know what was going on. We'd just have to watch him and wait to see what developed.

We sat on the floor in his room and read a few books, but he didn't want as many as usual and allowed himself to be put in his crib without any protest. A thought tickled me as I walked down the stairs. This wasn't the way I'd wanted it to be, but perhaps I could get her closer to home until Willie was well.

Jeff wasn't home from the hospital yet, and rather than call him, I dialed the answering service for the pediatrics practice and asked who was on call. There was a one-in-three chance that it would be Hugh, and the odds were with me that evening.

"Hugh, Willie has a fever," I told him when he returned my call. I could picture him rolling his eyes. When would it end with this family, he must have wondered. But he said nothing more than "Uh huh" and waited to hear more.

"Nothing serious, probably," I continued. "He doesn't have any other symptoms, but I don't want to bring Sarah home and expose her to whatever it is." I paused. "She is scheduled to be discharged from Baystate tomorrow." He knew that. "Do you think we can admit her to Franklin until Willie is better?"

"I think that can be arranged," he said, and we talked through the plan.

Funny how little I remember about the following day. I don't recall who stayed at home with Willie and his fever. Nothing about the drive to Baystate sticks in my mind. I don't remember gathering Sarah's mobile or her singing yellow bird or her "diamond ring" or any of the parapher-nalia we had strung on her crib to decorate her home-away-from-home. I don't remember dressing her. In contrast to the vivid picture I have of the outfit Sarah wore on the day she was admitted to the hospital, what she wore on the day of her discharge is a blank. All I recall of the discharge process is the pump nurse handing me a small metal instru-ment. Trying to figure it out, I turned it over in my hand.

"Bulldog clamp," he defined it. "If anything happens to her central line . . ." He left the rest unsaid while he demonstrated how to place the clamp on the tubing close to where it protruded from the dressing at Sarah's neck. The central IV line was sewn into a large vein that led to the heart. If the plastic tubing that came from the IV were cut, torn, pulled out, or accidentally traumatized in a fall or a car accident, it would be like slicing open a vein with a scalpel. Her blood would flow out from the vein like water flowing from the kitchen faucet.

I stuck my hand in my left front pants pocket and checked for holes. Then I slipped the clamp into the pocket. I patted it every now and again, just to be sure.

I don't remember saying good-bye to the floor nurses on that last day at Baystate. Sarah had been on the pediatric floor for seven days, and with rotating shifts and days off, the staff had changed from day to day. Except for Janice, who'd done the dressing change on the previous day, I hadn't come to know any of them very well. The real good-byes had taken place a week earlier in the pediatric ICU, where Marianne and the other nurses had bestowed a lifetime of blessings upon Sarah as her crib rolled out through the double doors.

While preparing for the discharge, the social worker who was organizing things asked whether I thought Sarah would need an ambulance for her transfer to the Franklin Medical Center. That seemed unnecessary. Since the original plan had been for me to drive her directly home from Baystate, I saw no reason not to drive her to Greenfield myself.

I don't remember walking out of the hospital, don't remember driving the car up to get the baby at the door, don't remember who held her while I did those things. What I do remember is the driving. I can see Sarah in her car seat beside me, and I remember how weirdly familiar it felt to have her there as I drove north on the highway and how my eyes kept drifting to the right. If I didn't peek under the blankets to look for the tubing and the gauze and the tape, she looked no different than she had on the day she had been admitted to the hospital in August.

I don't remember driving into the lot at the Franklin Medical Center, if someone met us at the emergency entrance, or if I carried her to the pediatrics floor. How can it all be a blank? Not even a blur but completely erased. I don't remember if Jeff joined us there. I have no recollection of how long Willie was sick or who stayed with him at the house on such short notice.

It was as if when the time came to stop worrying about whether the baby would live or die, my brain drowned itself in a blessed amnesia. I was able to move into a purely functioning mode, putting on my shoes and socks in the morning without having to mistrust where our lives might be when I dropped my clothing on the closet floor that night.

Sarah was in the hospital for a few days while Willie was sick, but I don't remember how many. And it seems inconceivable, but I don't remember even one thing about the day she came home from Franklin Medical Center for the last time.

What I do remember is an autumn of amazing beauty, spectacular even for New England. Light bounced off the leaves of the maple tree right outside our back door, and when I shuffled in to make coffee in the morning, I'd find the kitchen bathed in yellow. There are a few special days in October, some years more and some years fewer, when the colors in our house are transformed as if an interior decorator repaints the walls. Even the air changes hue. In October of 1986, it seemed that each day competed with the previous one in an all-natural beauty contest.

After Jeff kissed us goodbye each day, Sarah, Willie, and I reinvented ourselves as a threesome in the kitchen. Actually we were four, if you counted Miss Weed, who still sat at attention by Willie's high chair three times a day. Sarah perched in the infant seat I placed on the kitchen counter. Routine activities took us through the day, and the sun moved from east to west in a sky that was rarely touched by a cloud. Changing the colors in the house from morning gold to late afternoon crimson, the light seemed to move across the color wheel as the hours in the day slipped by. Sarah moved from cradle to bath, from counter top to a quilt on the floor. Wherever she went, the green lights of the apnea monitor flashed out the reassuring rhythm of her breathing.

All of that I remember.

While Sarah was in Franklin Medical Center those few days, I planned what I hoped would be a smooth routine for us when she came home. Willie could still go to Lynda's three mornings a week. That gave me time to do errands and keep the house organized, and he would have playtime with other kids. I would pick him up at lunchtime, and then he would head upstairs for his afternoon nap. Sarah could have much of her treatment while Willie slept, and that way we weren't tied down for the entire day if we had other things to do.

On the day of the first treatment, the pump nurse came to the house to help me and to answer questions about the procedure. I needed space to spread things out, and since Sarah wasn't rolling over yet, I set her up in the center of the queen-sized bed. She was not bothered by the activity. Most likely everything seemed both new and familiar. On my bedside stand I had arranged a supply of needles and syringes and all the equipment I needed for the treatment and dressing changes.

Once Sarah was in place, I diluted the medication. Amphotericin came as a powdery cake in a small glass vial. It had to be reconstituted with sterile water so it could be given intravenously. I added the medication to sixty cc (two ounces) of D5W, sterile water with a small amount of dextrose in it. That mixture had to be infused slowly over four hours. The pump was easy enough to use. I inserted the syringe with the medication into the pump and attached the tubing to Sarah's central line, which I had disinfected. I punched a few buttons similar to those on the front of a microwave oven, and the pump started to hum. I wrapped the tubing in foil so the medication would not be exposed to light, and we were in business.

Of course Sarah did not like having her IV dressing changed at home any more than she had in the hospital, and Jeff and I had to perform the ritual every other day. I knew Jeff would be the quicker of the two of us, so he did the dressing change. After positioning Sarah on the bed to accommodate my left-handed skills and Jeff's dominant right, I would gather her two hands in my right one and then turn her head towards her left shoulder. I held her head there with my left hand in order to fully expose her neck. When she was immobilized, Jeff went to work.

He was all business during the procedure while I did the sympathetic cooing. He peeled the paper tape from her neck and chest and lifted the old gauze from around the IV line. Considering how bulky and complicated her neck looked when it was dressed, the actual IV site was simple and clean. A spaghetti-sized white catheter exited from the skin behind her right ear, but the tiny tube threaded under the skin for about two inches to a place where it actually entered a vein. The distance prevented bacteria from entering the major vein. One black suture held the catheter in place.

While Jeff, all concentration, swabbed the skin behind Sarah's ear with Betadine solution, I tried to distract her. But after weeks of hospital dressing changes, this baby knew what was going on, and she didn't like it. Holding her still was not as easy as it might seem. She weighed only nine pounds, but she was quite strong in the conviction that she was being wronged. Feeling disloyal, I could not help smiling at her miniature fury. I was amused at her scrunched-up face and kicking legs, and I rejoiced at her feistiness. Occasionally Jeff would let us know he could hear her. "Ahhh, quitchyer fussin'," he would growl, never flustered by the crying, never changing the pace of his precise movements. Then, after he was done with the cutting, taping, and putting her all back together like a diminutive Humpty Dumpty, he would lift her from the bed, wipe away the teardrops from her cheeks, and cover her salty face with kisses. She would perch upright in his arms, re-evaluating her world and forgiving us once again.

Finally, in mid-October, the days of amphotericin b therapy were nearly accomplished. I called Barbara Stechenberg to find out how we should officially end the treatment and who would remove the central line. It seemed weird that the whole thing would just stop. One day I was carefully mixing, measuring, and calibrating. The next, would I do nothing more than settle my baby for an afternoon nap?

Dr. Stechenberg, bless her heart, seemed to understand that I needed some kind of closure to Sarah's saga, a finale that would tie hospital and home together.

Physicians from Baystate came to the Franklin Medical Center several times each month to teach continuing education classes to local doctors. In some fortuitous confluence, the pediatric presenter for October of that year happened to be Barbara Stechenberg.

Dr. Stechenberg said I did not have to drive Sarah to Springfield to take the catheter out. No, I did not have to take Sarah to the Franklin, either. And no, she did not want Hugh or Jeff, though either was quite capable, to pull the catheter.

She said, "Kathryn and I will come to your house after the lecture on Friday." Kathryn was the pediatric chief resident and had taken care of Sarah in September. "We'll be there at 10:30." I looked at the calendar. On Friday morning Willie was scheduled to be at Lynda's, and I wouldn't have to worry about him during the procedure. The timing was perfect.

"You're the doctor," I said, and because I'd found ten pounds of forgotten blueberries in my freezer that morning, I promised her a co-pay of homemade blueberry muffins.

I mused over the doctors' impending house call. How like women, I thought, allowing myself a moment to dwell in unabashedly sexist thoughts, to want to see Sarah's story through to the very end. I knew the male physicians who had taken care of Sarah were every bit as invested in the outcome of her story as were these two women, but I didn't think the male doctors had the same need to actually be there for what we hoped would be the last medical moment in Sarah's first year. Jeff certainly didn't. He would have pulled the catheter without a blink if I'd let him. He would have let Hugh pull it and been happy if I told him about it when he got home from work at the end of the day. But I had the distinct feeling that it was different for Barbara Stechenberg and that it was almost as important for her to be a part of this moment as it was for me to have her there.

The doctors used the kitchen counter as their treatment table. They were just a few feet down from where the griddle was usually set up for Sunday morning pancakes although there hadn't been many pancake breakfasts since January. The counter was at a convenient height for them as they stood to do their work. I covered the Formica surface with towels, topped the towels with a flannel receiving blanket, and then laid Sarah down on top of the layers. I had removed her shirt so the doctors could get to her neck, and although she looked wary as I put her flat, she did not cry. The two doctors competed for Sarah's attentions, and she was too fascinated by the strangers to fuss the way she would have with Jeff and me.

Doctor Kathryn slipped her hands into a pair of gloves and began to pry the tape from Sarah's neck and chest. She gently removed the dressing, exposing the skin. Doctor Barbara held Sarah's hands and kept her entertained as Kathryn removed the dressing. I was extraneous, just an observer this time. When the tape was off and the gauze removed, leaving only skin and catheter, Kathryn used a small pair of pointed sterile scissors to snip the one suture that held the catheter in place. Then she stopped, and looked at her mentor. The veteran doctor nodded and said, "Go ahead. You do it."

With quick fingers Kathryn pinched the exposed end of the catheter and swept the rest of its four inches out from under Sarah's skin where it had dwelled as a lifeline for almost three months. Kathryn held it up for all to see, and the white tip boinged crazily in the air like an unruly hair in a cowlick. The three adults cheered.

Sarah was still flat on her back. Her eyes were wide and seemed surprised. She looked as if she might have something to say, but then decided she was not upset when it was all over. Dr. Barbara, keeping up a constant chatter directed at Sarah, continued to envelop the two small hands in her own. Sarah stared at her doctor warily, not yet convinced that she should smile while Kathryn held a gauze pad firmly over the hole in Sarah's skin where the catheter had been. After the required minutes of pressure to the site, Kathryn fastened the last bit of gauze in place with a piece of tape and sat the baby up. Appearing a little shell-shocked, Sarah looked around the room. Free at last.

The coffee pot ceased gurgling, and we moved to the dining room table. With their work done, the doctors took time to look out the windows and notice the colors that bathed the room. It was another in that unbroken string of sunny October days, and shades of yellows and oranges and reds were brilliant. From the vantage point of Barbara Stechenberg's generous lap, Sarah lost her dazed look and moved her green eyes from one to the other of us. She watched intently as we passed a basketful of blueberry muffins around the table. I poured coffee, and for all of the celebrating we were doing, the coffee may as well have had bubbles in it. It didn't matter. We raised our steaming mugs and said, "To Sarah!"

HO! HO! HO!

Soon after Willie's birth, Muz and Puz had given us a video camera. We did not take any movies of Sarah in the hospital although eventually I wished we had. By the time Christmas of 1986 arrived, however, the tide had changed, and the video camera's red light was on for some event nearly every day. I recorded any sight or sound that threatened to be cute.

The camera ran in Pennsylvania where we'd celebrated the first part of Christmas with the Blomstedts. Jeff's brothers and sisters were home for the holidays. His nephews, Eric and little Jeffrey, were ten and six years old, and Willie was awestruck by his cousins. Puz was in the midst of chemotherapy and radiation treatments and dealing with their side effects, but he put forth his best effort to participate in the holiday.

One evening Muz shooed Jeff and me out for a dinner date—she'd made reservations for us to go to a local inn for dinner. We hadn't been out for an evening together since Sarah's return home. Sarah was still attached to the apnea monitor, and the only babysitting we trusted was the respite nurse. We received respite nursing care for a few hours each month. We ended up having a nurse come on Friday afternoons, and Jeff and I went to see the therapist my friend Barbara had recommended to me during the summer. As I came to realize, we personified the crisis theory I'd learned about in college. Jeff and I had weathered the year, but we'd each experienced Sarah's birth and hospitalization in our own way. After Sarah came home in October, we realized we needed help figuring out what had happened and where the experience left us as a couple and a family. By December, I could actually see how we might be stronger as a result of our work with the therapist. So Muz's instincts were right. Though we preferred her cooking to any chef's, it was good for us to have some time alone. At the inn we enjoyed a glass of wine, perfect crab cakes, a fire in the hearth, and festive holiday decorations. But like many couples out on their first dates after having a child, we mostly talked about the kids.

When we returned to the Chadds Ford home after dinner, white candles still shone in the windows, but the house was settled for the night. Muz, in her robe and slippers, leaned against the kitchen counter and told us Sarah had spent much of the evening on a blanket on the living room floor, and Puz had been down there with her. "He was all done in," Muz said. He'd gone to bed soon after the little ones were down.

As Puz ate his pancakes the next morning, he described the antics of his grandchildren with wry delight and wondered, as he had many times, how he and Muz could possibly have had the energy to raise five children of their own. "Somehow, they just snuck up on us," he said, shaking his head. Sarah and Willie have no memory of that last Christmas with their grandfather, but I always think of the evening they spent with Puz as the best of all the holiday gifts.

The next location for the 1986 holiday film documentary was in Enfield with the LaScala family. In the footage taken on the Christmas day when Sarah was eleven months old, she sat on the lap of my mother's sister Ann. Whether the camera was on or off, Auntie Ann's arms were wrapped around the baby all of that Christmas afternoon. Fortunately my mother was so busy being hostess that she didn't have much time for baby holding. Otherwise we would have needed the wisdom of King Solomon to convince the sisters that they must share the baby.

Sarah was, of course, too young to care much about Christmas gifts. She observed the holiday activities from the safety of her great aunt's lap. Sarah paid close attention to the most interesting action in the room: her brother and cousin Stephen. The boys darted around the room as if glued together at the elbows. They ran from a giant puzzle to wooden train sets to yellow construction vehicles. Sarah wore a bright green jumper over a white blouse in a kind of Swiss miss look. Someone stuck a silver bow on the top of her head, and it wobbled as her attention moved from the boys to her grandma and then to Santa Claus, who arrived in the midst of much commotion and sounded suspiciously familiar as he swept into the living room with a red sack full of gifts.

"Ho, ho, ho!" Santa boomed. "Are there any kids in this house? I have some presents here for kids, but I'm in a big hurry! Is there a Stephen here? And a Willie? What about a Sarah? HO! HO! HO! There they are, one, two, three! Merrrrrrrry Christmas, everybody!" And then he was gone, leaving a pile of gifts and three wide-eyed children in his wake.

The family was gathered in my parents' living room, and when it was time for gift-giving, Mom stood in front of the Christmas tree and called for everyone's attention. She drew herself up to her full five feet and two inches, cleared her throat, and began reading from a sheet of lined paper. When she finished her poem, she wended her way through the gifts the boys had strewn on the living room floor and picked up a large, wrapped box. Then she turned to Jeff and handed the box to him.

Accepting it with a hug, Jeff resumed his seat, slipped the ribbons off, and tore the paper from the box. He peered inside.

"Oh . . . my . . . goodness," he said, separating each word. "What is this?"

Reaching into the box, Jeff took out face paints, a plastic package containing a bulbous red nose that squeaked when he squeezed it, and a bright red wig.

"What is this?" he repeated again, smiling but mystified. There was more. Finally he threw back his head and laughed, and the rest of the family, who overflowed the room's sofas and chairs, craned to see.

From the box he started to pull what looked like yards and yards of multicolored fabric. It seemed to emerge endlessly. When completely unfolded and held up to Jeff's front, the fabric revealed itself to be a white, one-piece coverall dotted with half-dollar-sized spots of yellow, red, green, and blue. It was long enough to cover Jeff's six-foot-two-inch frame and wide enough to fit him and a friend inside its seams. Everyone applauded Mom, complimenting her on her clever, hand-made gift and for having given it to exactly the right person.

HAPPY BIRTHDAY

Three weeks later, on January 12, 1987, I walked into the Franklin Medical Center with Sarah in my arms and found a clown in the hall near the emergency room. Wondering if it was okay to stare, patients and staff walked past him and grinned uncertainly. I turned Sarah around, her back against my front, so that we both could face the clown. She viewed him from the safety of my arms. I walked closer, and he composed himself. Then he spoke to her quietly.

"Hello, Sarah Tate!" (That was Willie's way of saying Sarah Kate, the nickname we'd all adopted when she came home.) "Don't you look pretty in your pink dress."

Sarah stared at the clown. He reached out and squeezed one little white shoe. "Do you know who I am?"

Face to face, she studied him without blinking, without smiling, apparently mystified by the sound of a familiar voice coming out of a visage of white pancake makeup surrounded by a red halo.

Sarah's birthday party was about to begin.

How could we possibly celebrate the day? Jeff and I puzzled over that question in the weeks before January 12. We had much to be grateful for, and only a fireworks display could come near to declaring what Sarah's birthday meant to us. When we thought about the many people at both hospitals who had followed her progress, celebrated her successes and worried over her setbacks, we realized that Sarah's first birthday was not the year for a quiet family party. This birthday celebration needed to include everyone.

More people gathered around the clown and the baby. With the help of one of the impromptu party guests, I slipped a marble sheet cake out of its box. It was decorated with a bunch of colored-frosting balloons and the words, Happy Birthday Sarah. I organized the cake, cups, cider, and napkins on a stainless steel surgical cart commandeered for the occasion. While I cut cake, Jeff distributed slices to the small gathering that surrounded us. When that group dispersed, I took the baby from the nurse who'd been holding her, Jeff grabbed the cart, and we started our pilgrimage through the hospital.

Every time we went around a corner, staff, patients, and visitors stopped. They looked. It was the clown, of course, giving them pause. The clown would say something indicating that he knew the nurse, the cafeteria woman, or the patient, and surprise would change to laughter and laughter to surprise again when they realized who the clown was and who the baby was. "Oh! It's Dr. B's baby!" They cooed and oohed and touched her dress, her shoes, her hands. Sarah's birthday dress was pink and trimmed with white lace. She wore white tights and soft white baby shoes. She sat up like a sentry in my arms, and though she hadn't taken her usual nap that afternoon, she did not fuss.

Sarah weighed twelve pounds on her first birthday. Her hair was a fine, dark brown. The little berry of a hemangioma was shrinking and less obvious as it receded into her hair. Her face was full, and her green eyes were alert as they watched her visitors and followed the clown. The strength of her neck muscles was uneven due to the position she'd had to maintain with the central line in place, and she held her head at a slight tilt. It made her look a bit quizzical as if she were considering a thought. Sarah obviously considered the party a serious event, and she didn't smile much that afternoon.

Though we'd started dispensing cake on the ground floor near the ER, we officially began the party on the top floor of the hospital. The obstetrical unit on the third floor was where the medical part of our experience had started a year earlier. We came through the elevator doors, and I handed Sarah to Jill, the head nurse who'd admitted Sarah to the nursery back in April. Jill was obviously itching to get her hands on the baby. Leaving them to get reacquainted, I walked over to peek into the large room where the nurses usually observed women in early labor. I couldn't help but look up reflexively at the televisions suspended from the ceiling. I half-expected to see a football game in progress, but the screens were blank, and the room was empty and silent. I stood for a moment, alone, thinking about all the stories that started in that room.

One year later the action was taking place in the hallway, and I returned to where the clown handed out cake and cider to the obstetrics nurses. Sarah was in somebody else's arms by then. Since Jeff knew these people and seemed to have things under control, I wandered in another direction. I peered through the nursery windows at the new babies wrapped like pink and blue sausages in their receiving blankets. Sarah had never made it to that room as a newborn.

After saying goodbye to the OB and nursery staff, we progressed through the hospital, one floor at a time. We visited each unit, and in every one the staff first smiled at the clown then melted when they recognized the baby. Jeff cut more squares of cake and pressed them on anyone who would take them. The nurses took a moment to admire the baby and nibble on cake.

Our final destination was the pediatrics floor. Though this was not where Sarah had spent her most critical time, the pediatric nurses knew her well. When we arrived there, it was change of shift, and we managed to catch both day and evening staff. The nurses took her from my arms and passed her around, marveling, "Look at how big you are! Look at those pretty eyes! You are so beautiful!" Not fussy but not smiling, either, Sarah absorbed the attention.

By the time our rounds were finished, the cake had been reduced to a few sad pieces and a smattering of crumbs, the clown's makeup was a little smudged, and we had a tired baby on our hands. We cleaned up our mess and gathered the accoutrements of our party-on-wheels. Jeff walked out into the cold January afternoon air with me to fill the car with the things that would come home.

"I'll go check on things in the dialysis unit," he said. "I'm not even going to change. I'll be home in a little while." At that moment, the clown looked as tired as the baby.

It was nearly four o'clock when I pointed the car out of the hospital parking lot. It was time to get Willie. I looked over at Sarah, her eyes glassy from fatigue and over-stimulation. No wonder she was tired. She had missed her nap, and even before the hospital party she had presided over a cupcake party with Willie and all the kids at Lynda's. I knew she'd be asleep before we reached the first traffic light. I thought about the date again. At this moment one year ago, where had I been? On a stretcher at the entrance to Baystate, staring at the ceiling, more dumbfounded than afraid. As Jeff and I had been swept into the current that would carry us through the year, I'd assumed that when this date came around again it would conjure up feelings of sadness and pain. But the brush with tragedy had done just the opposite. January 12 had been transformed into a holiday.

IT TAKES A LOT OF LOVE
TO MAKE A POUND

The staff at Franklin Medical Center had followed Sarah's progress, cared for her as their patient, and worried over Jeff for a year. We loved them for that. But our larger debt of gratitude belonged to the people in Springfield who had taken care of Sarah from the moment of her birth and through each medical crisis. On the day after Sarah's birthday party in Greenfield, the way-back of the car was again taken over by a balloon-frosted cake and a cooler that held a few cartons of vanilla ice cream. We were on our way to another party.

As we passed through Greenfield, I turned around to check out what was happening in the back seat and saw Sarah's eyes already closed. Willie had started the trip in an upright position but was fighting his own heavy eyelids. Within a few minutes his head lolled to one side. I told Jeff to adjust the rearview mirror so he could see the passengers behind us, and he smiled at the view. Nap time in the car. A golden hour. I reached over and took Jeff's right hand and squeezed it. He smiled again. I fell back into my seat and let my eyes close.

My thoughts turned to the people we were going to visit. How often do the staff see their babies after they left the hospital? I wondered. What are they expecting from Sarah?

By her first birthday, Sarah was not doing things a one-year-old would normally do. She was twelve months old biologically but only eight months old developmentally. Doctor Hugh said not to worry; Sarah would follow her own schedule for a while. Her smile remained toothless. She wasn't walking yet. She wasn't crawling either though she would tentatively rock on her hands and knees a few times each day. When I put her down in one spot, she would be in the same place fifteen minutes later, playing with whatever toy I'd placed in front of her. If the pediatrician said she was okay, Sarah's lack of mobility suited me just fine, especially when I followed Willie from room to room, trying to save him from self-destruction.

It seemed as if I had just closed my eyes when I felt the car slow down. Jeff was turning off the highway. My thoughts dispersed in a kind of mist, and I recognized the familiar intersection. We had arranged for my mother to meet us in Baystate's parking lot, and she was already there. Jeff unbuckled the safety belt from the car seat containing the slumbering Willie and moved the entire package from our back seat to

Grandma's. She peeked in at Sarah, gave hugs to Jeff and me, and said she'd have dinner ready for us when we arrived in Enfield after the party.

Jeff drove up to the curb in front of the NICU entrance to the medical center and stopped the car. I gathered the baby from her seat and stepped onto the curb. Jeff moved the car to a parking space and joined us on the sidewalk with cake, ice cream, and party paraphernalia. Then we walked through the familiar doors into the hospital.

How odd it was to wave casually to the guard and say, "We're just going up to the NICU to visit. They're expecting us . . ." How strange to walk with light steps over the linoleum-tiled corridor that once seemed so gloomy, to move as anonymously as the other visitors down the hallway. We passed interns and residents who wore stethoscopes around their necks and harried looks on their faces and who looked even younger than they had the year before. Jeff and I were loaded down with baby and party goods, yet it seemed my feet hardly touched the floor. It was a dreamy feeling, kind of like being in the middle of a wavy oasis that appears far down a black road on a ninety-degree summer afternoon.

Press the button. Wait for the elevator. Step in, the two of us and the baby. Feel the lurch as the elevator moves. The baby watches with bright eyes.

"Bing!" The number five lights up overhead. Step off the elevator. See the double doors. Punch the big round button that opens them. "Open, Sesame!" I allow myself to think, just for the fun of it.

We did no hand-scrubbing at the sinks on that day. Just a peek and a knock at the window to let Beverly, the NICU's nursing director, know we were there. She was my college classmate. I waved to her and said, "Hi, Beverly," into the window. "We're back."

Beverly was on the phone but nodded, smiled, and pointed us toward the staff's break room. I'd never been there before, but it looked like the break room of every hospital unit I'd seen. A disheveled mess of unwashed coffee cups and open textbooks sat on a central table surrounded by chairs that were probably never pushed in, and pairs of clogs and scuffed white shoes with lopsided heels lay in a corner near the lockers.

We had a few minutes to get organized, so I cleared the table and took the cake out of its box. I stuck the Number 1 candle in the white frosting.

When staff members began to filter in, the room lit up and the mess receded into the background. Suddenly the faces we'd known, all smiling, surrounded us. The doctors and nurses hugged Jeff and me, exclaimed over Sarah, talked to each other. I kept thinking something about them seemed different, a little unfamiliar, and I finally realized what it was. In the months we'd spent in the NICU, we rarely saw these people smile. It was odd to see them happy. Sarah was immediately snatched from Jeff by one of the smiling people and began her travels around the room.

A few days before the parties, I'd found a hair decoration that seemed made just for this birthday. It was a bow of pink satin trimmed with white lace that measured barely an inch across. The backing was plastic with a Velcro clasp. In the morning, after I'd dressed her, I'd twisted a tuft of her hair into a ponytail on the top of her head and Velcroed the miniature bow there. Observing her at the party through the eyes of her caregivers, I saw an adorable, bright-eyed, happy baby with a silly tuft of hair standing on the top of her head. Tears sprang to my eyes.

She was more engaged than she had been the day before. Maybe the Franklin party had been good practice for her, and she was more used to the socializing. Maybe the clown had made her feel she had to be extra vigilant at the Franklin. Or maybe she just needed the pre-party nap in the car. Whatever the reason, she was generous with her smiles for the NICU staff as they gathered around her in a great cluster. If her doctors' smiles were unfamiliar to us, Sarah's smile had been nonexistent when they knew her, so they did everything they could to keep it going. I watched as Dr. Meyer, the neonatologist who was present at Sarah's birth, bent forward to talk with Sarah as she held court from the arms of one of her nurses. I thought of the first mew that came from Sarah on the night of her birth and dabbed at my eyes with a napkin as the same baby, one year later, rewarded Kathy Meyer with waving arms and a goofy smile.

There was a wealth of intelligence in that room on that afternoon, but the group of educated professionals was suddenly reduced to a grinning bunch of adults who sang "Happy Birthday" with a remarkable lack of musical talent. By then Sarah was back with me, facing the cake and all of her friends. She kicked her feet with the excitement of the moment, and her smile twinkled and spread over the room like pixie dust.

A few days after the birthday visit, I went to the store to pick up the birthday and holiday pictures. When I got home, I spread them on the kitchen counter. There were many shots of the Christmas scene with my family in Enfield and then the more sedate version of the holiday we had celebrated in Pennsylvania with the Blomstedts. At the bottom of the pile, I found the birthday collection, and the very last photo was one from the NICU on Sarah's birthday. I stared at the image. Sarah, thumb planted in her mouth, sits in the arms of another Sarah, the NICU's clinical nurse specialist. Standing to the right and a little behind is Dr. Gary Rockwell, who had been Sarah's attending physician for the month of January. Next to him is David, Sarah's primary nurse, and then Dr. Meyer. On the left are two nurses, Denise, back to work part-time after delivering her own baby earlier in the year, and Lauren, who took care of Sarah on David's days off, the ones I had begrudged him. I took the photo at the end of the afternoon, and Sarah was staring into space by that time, her eyes slightly glazed. The rest of the group smiled broadly. I wanted to hug all of those people again.

I took the NICU birthday photograph over to the cabinet where we kept our photo albums and found the one that documented the first year of Sarah's life. I flipped to the back of the book and found a blank page. After pulling back the clear magnetic cover, I eyeballed the dimensions of the page and stuck the group photo that commemorated Sarah's birthday right in the center. The final page of the album would hold a picture of the intrepid Sarah Katherine Blomstedt with the people who had been her dedicated caregivers and unflagging cheerleaders. That image of Sarah, surrounded by just a few representatives of those who had contributed to her survival, would be the last one of her in the hospital.

Finally, we could close the book.

EPILOGUE:
MARCH 12, 2003

I don't even bother to use my signal light as I make a right hand turn into Lynda's driveway. At ten in the morning the country road that extends behind and in front of me has no other car on it. We are having an unusually snowy winter, even by New England standards, and Lynda's yard is completely white, so the collection of toys and kids' equipment is not spread about the way I had been used to seeing it. The house looks the same, the barn-red siding in good shape, and the only way I can measure how much time has passed since I've been here to pick up my preschool children is the size of the white pines that border the driveway. They are no longer sparse and spindly but stand tall and upright, tufted branches ruffling in March wind.

When I open the car door, I find that droplets sprinkling my windshield have become icy specks bouncing on the hard blacktop of the driveway and ticking through pine needles. As I pull up the hood of my coat and prepare to make a dash for the house, the kitchen's storm door opens and Sarah pokes the upper half of her body out the door and around the railing. Even from this distance, I can see that her smile is a little sheepish, a little something else.

"Don't come in, Mom!" she hollers through the sleet, her dark pony tail swinging to the side as she leans into the air.

I stop where I am though my face is being stung by hot-cold needles. "Okay, I won't," I call back. "I just wanted to say hi to Lynda."

"I'll be out in a minute."

Sarah disappears into the house. I am semi-aware, as I turn back to the car, that something about Lynda's house is different. Ah . . . the porch is new, a proper landing zone for kids with wet boots who, in our days here, clomped onto a rectangle of rug at the entry to the kitchen. Now, on the portico above the porch, a crescent moon sits at a jaunty angle surrounded by white stars. Lynda's house is still a place of enchantment. I want to go in. I want to smell banana bread.

Instead, I run around the car and slide into the front seat on the passenger side. I turn the key in the ignition and fiddle with the tape player, going back to my recorded book. When I look up again, Lynda is on the porch, waving to me. Her hair has gone completely white since the last time I saw her. I eject the tape and roll the window down.

"Hi, Susan," she yells above the din of falling sleet. "I didn't want you to think I was being unsociable." As if Lynda could be. She's drying her hands on a towel and looking around. "Hey, what's it doing out here?"

Above the din of the precipitation, we exchange a few sentences as we do every few years when we run into one another. Then Lynda disappears behind her door, and soon Sarah is running down the driveway, ducking her head in an attempt to avoid the heavenly assault.

She makes a face when she arrives at the passenger door and sees me there. Sarah is supposed to be doing the driving. She was hoping I'd forget. She is seventeen and has had her permit for a year but has been too busy to take driving lessons. Now I insist that she drive whenever we are in the car together. Even if she chooses not to get her license for a while, it's all about practice.

So, she runs over to the other side of the car, opens the door, and plops into the driver's seat, smoothing the icy droplets out of her dark hair. We click our seatbelt buckles simultaneously.

"How is it going?" I ask. It is a rhetorical question. I know I won't get a real answer because what Sarah is doing at Lynda's is a surprise. For me. She and Jeff have concocted some sort of mischief. I discovered there was a mysterious project going on when she had transportation problems and I ended up having to be her driver when Jeff couldn't do it.

In the years after our kids went off to elementary school, Lynda has become the local expert in paper maché. She teaches workshops in her home and at local schools. Both Sarah and Will created various critters under Lynda's tutelage. Sarah started in the fourth grade with a chimpanzee holding a banana in one hand, moved on to a gray wolf when she was in her fifth-grade, endangered-species phase, and then created a bright green tree frog for her sixth grade science fair project. Will's first work was a fisher in its white winter coat, and in 1994, the year after Miss Weed passed away, Will spent months working on a life-sized golden retriever he gave to Jeff for his forty-sixth birthday. So I suspect that I am getting something in paper maché, but beyond that I can't even begin to guess.

Sarah adjusts the mirrors and driver's seat and then turns her head to look over her right shoulder, the pupils of her green eyes dilated with the attention she devotes to perfecting this new skill.

"I don't have to turn the wheel or anything, do I?" she asks. I look behind me just to be sure. The driveway is long and straight.

"No," I say, trying not to smile. "Just hold it on course. You may need to make little adjustments to stay straight."

She backs out to the road competently, puts the gearshift in drive, and turns us east on Boyle Road.

"She is so sweet," Sarah says, her eyes trained on the road ahead, referring now to Lynda. Sarah smiles, and her eyes crinkle in the corners when she does. "When I was getting ready to leave, Lynda said to me, 'Do you have your coat and boots and gloves?' just like when I was a little kid. Just like a second mom."

"I think she is one of the nicest people I have ever known," I say out loud and allow myself to get a little sentimental about Lynda, the way her path has woven in and out of our lives for the past seventeen years.

We pass the Gill Elementary School on our left. No kids are outside at recess today. On Main Road I see a field of Holstein cows that seem unfazed by the sleet drumming on their hides. We go by the fire station and I notice a police car sitting there. I think of all the places that I would point out to Willie in those sad days, those sharp-pain days, when I was torn in half, glad to have my little boy back for the day but already miserable with the worry of what might have happened to my little girl in the hour since I'd left her. Now Sarah, the same Sarah who had been at the center of all that worry, I have to remind myself, is driving me home from Lynda's house. Sometimes I have to pinch myself.

When Will was learning to drive, I wasn't allowed to say anything when I was in the front seat because he thought he already knew everything. When Sarah drives, I usually try to make small talk in order to have her get used to a little bit of distraction. Otherwise she drives with locked-on concentration, rarely saying a word except to ask an occasional question: "Can I go now?" or "Is this where I turn?" Sarah and her brother are a study in opposites. Will from Gill, as he is called by the girls on the sidelines of the soccer field, was six feet, five inches tall the last time I checked. Sarah is five feet and one inch. He weighs one hundred ninety pounds. She is that minus the ninety. He is calm and unflappable, dubbed Mr. Steady by his soccer coach when he was in the fifth grade, and the name still fits. Sarah is intense and always wants to do things E-X-A-C-T-L-Y-R-I-G-H-T. We have called her Miss Rules from the time she was four years old, the perfectly behaved child who never had to sit in timeout in school.

They summed themselves up one morning at breakfast. It must have been a Thursday, because they were eating French toast and that was our Thursday standard. Often breakfasts before school were silent, but on this morning the talk was about sports.

Sarah, stabbing at a square of French toast: "Do you know what I hate the most?"

I was putting dishes away. "What?" I asked.

Sarah, swirling the square round and round in a puddle of syrup: "I hate when the coach lectures us for ten minutes about everything we have to do in the game and then says, 'Now just go out there and have fun.'"

Will, working over his plate with knife and fork: "What's wrong with that?"

"IT IS NOT FUN!" She speaks in capital letters, but she can't really yell. One of her vocal cords is paralyzed from having been on a ventilator for so long, and her voice is soft and a little hoarse. But she still manages to emphasize: "IT'S HARD WORK OUT THERE."

She might complain over breakfast on the morning before a game when her stomach is full of butterflies, but she knows and we know that she wouldn't spend her time any other way. When she applied to Loomis Chaffee School for tenth grade admission, one of the questions on the form asked which sports she liked to play and which was her favorite. Her answers: "In the fall, field hockey. In the winter, squash. In the spring, lacrosse." I couldn't bear to tell her that what they were asking was, "Of the sports you play, pick the one that is your favorite." Whatever the sport was for the season, that was her favorite. Picking one would be like asking parents which of their children they love the best. They love all of them, each in a different way.

Will stops cutting his French toast and shakes his head. His shoulders are also shaking, the way they do when he laughs.

"Why don't I have any of that?" he asks, referring, I have to assume, to the fire that Sarah was spewing.

Will does what the coaches say to do. He really does have fun out there. He participates in three varsity sports, too: soccer, swimming, and crew. He plays hard with that big body, but he doesn't worry much about it before or after the contest. He gets out on the field or in the pool or in the boat, gives what he has to the team, has a great time, and leaves the sport behind when it is over. After more than one of his soccer games, I've seen Will stop in front of the net at the end of the field, throw his gym bag on the grass, and spend ten minutes playing goalie for the coach's two little sons. Pounding Will with shots on goal, they do their best to imitate the big boys. He finishes their games by wrestling and rolling on the ground with them for a few minutes. Then he saunters over to Jeff and me.

"Thanks for coming." He always says that, sounding a little formal. More often than not there are blood stains on the front of his lucky green tee shirt. He might ask what we are having for dinner, and he appears to think for a minute about whether he should come home for the meal or stay for the dining hall's entree. Although he is a day student at a boarding school, he usually chooses to stay. He says "I'll see you later" and begins the long walk across the field. After her games, on the other hand, Sarah processes plays, talks things over with Jeff, criticizes her performance, tries to figure out what went right, what went wrong, and what she can do better the next time.

Big and small. Boy and girl. Night and day. Yin and yang. A gallon of milk and six sticks of butter.

We continue the drive down Main Road, passing the houses of Sarah's former classmates and the women who are now my friends: friends who walk with me, friends who bike with me, friends who worked on the Gill School carnival with me, friends who can hardly stand knowing that we lived only minutes apart when Sarah was born. We met when our children started kindergarten together. These women wouldn't be my friends if Sarah hadn't survived. Now we walk our dogs—Miss Weed was followed by Sniffy, another golden retriever—through the woods in Gill and wish we had known one another when our kids were small.

By the time Sarah and I head down the long hill that brings us to the end of Main Road, the relentless, noisy sleet has turned to a soft rain. I didn't notice when it changed. The rhythm of the windshield wipers is steady now, clearing the blur away.

"Does the road seem slippery?" I ask her, breaking the silence.

"No. I think it's fine," she answers, her eyes focused on the pavement ahead.

We come to the intersection of Main Road and French King Highway. Sarah puts on the left-hand signal and waits for the light to change. Green for go.

We turn left and head for home.

A REALLY BIG CHART

a discussion of how the book *Small Wonder* was written
by Susan LaScala, FNP

When I started to write this story in 1997, I had only memories to work with. I had a calendar I'd scribbled on, but I didn't have the weights, times, or sequences of events, and I wanted to tell the story exactly the way it happened. I had vivid recollections of events from Sarah's first year but, of course, there were gaps. I hadn't kept a journal. Nor did I accumulate much memorabilia that year. Though I otherwise often have a camera in my hands, I hardly took a picture during Sarah's time in the hospital. If I couldn't be sure of a happy ending, I wasn't sure I wanted to remember anything at all.

So, I needed some facts. I called the medical records department at Baystate Medical Center. I asked the friendly voice at the other end of the line if I could get hospital records from 1986.

"I'll have to send you to the archives, Dear."

I went, via telephone, to the archives. I pictured a dark room in the bowels of Baystate Medical Center, torches illuminating the stairways. The next woman who answered the phone sounded quite modern, erasing the imaginary scene, and I repeated my request: I wanted my daughter's hospital records from 1986.

"No problem," she said.

"It is going to be a big chart," I said.

"That's not a problem," she said again.

"You don't understand," I said. "This is going to be a really big chart. She was in the hospital for nine months." I told her I didn't want all of the pages. I wanted the nurses' notes, the doctors' progress notes, and the daily vital sign sheets. I also wanted the x-ray and ultrasound reports. That was it. No social worker consultations, respiratory, or other therapies.

"Okay," said the woman. "The charge is twenty-five cents per page."

I gulped, but I gave her my name and address. She told me how to sign for a release of records, and she said it would probably take a week to get the copies to me.

An hour later the phone rang. It was the woman from the Baystate archives again. She sounded a little distressed.

"I, um, pulled the chart you asked for," she said. "But I just want to tell you. It's really big."

"I know. It must be huge," I said, smiling. "It's okay," I told her. "If you send me the parts I asked for, I think it will be manageable."

A week later a box came in the mail. In it were Sarah's records and a bill for $125.00. Five hundred pages. I brought the box into the kitchen and opened it. I picked up the top page and started to read.

Even with Sarah's medical records, I worried about writing the story honestly and factually. At first the nurse dominated the writer in me, and the nurse compelled me to write the story almost as if it were a medical record. My critics said that made for true but overly clinical storytelling. I felt uncomfortable writing about an event if I couldn't remember it clearly, but the memories were choppy, and I wasn't sure how to connect them. Then one day, while I sat at my computer, I heard something that allowed the nurse-writer to step back.

Usually when I sit down to write, I turn off radio and TV. On that afternoon I must have gone to the word processor without intending to stay, and the radio was still playing. While staring at the computer screen, I half-heard an ongoing conversation. Terry Gross, the host of *Fresh Air* on National Public Radio, was interviewing Daniel Schacter, the chairman of Harvard's Department of Psychology and a leading expert on memory. He was talking about his book, *The Seven Sins of Memory: How the Mind Forgets and Remembers*. I don't know why it caught my attention, but it was as if some divine power placed me within earshot of that conversation. I turned sideways in my chair and listened.

Dr. Schacter talked about the flaws and limitations of memory. In his book he discusses seven "sins" or weaknesses of memory in humans, but what captivated me, the nurse, was his discussion of the way hormonal systems are activated when humans are faced with frightening events. When adrenaline is released, the body is mobilized for action but the brain is also placed on alert. Memory for the experience is improved under the influence of adrenaline and cortisol. Well, no wonder, I thought. I'm sure if there were such a thing as an adrenaline meter and if I had plugged my finger into it in 1986, my adrenaline levels would have been elevated for some part of each day. Every time the phone rang my anxiety level spiked. Adrenaline probably factored into every meeting with a doctor, every lab result I waited for, every time I sped up or down the highway to or from one of my children. That adrenaline, frequently being released into my circulation, was one possible explanation for the strength of my memories from that year. But then I read about one of the sins Dr. Schacter describes: the sin of transience, forgetting that occurs with the passage of time. I may have remembered many incidents and details from that year, but with eleven years between the events and the writing, could the memories be accurate?

I have a photograph of Sarah at the age of three, sitting with Jeff on the flat roof over our kitchen. She holds a hammer in her right hand, and the hammer is poised over a nail that her brave father is holding in place. Some years later I was trying to remember a detail about renovations we had done to our house. As I ruminated on the building process, a rusty set of gears started turning in my head, and they connected my rendition of Sarah's birth story with the photograph. A flicker of consternation ran through me. Until those renovations were complete, our master bedroom had been on the first floor of the house, and only Willie's room and a guest room were upstairs. But I'd written about a moment in August 1986 when I walked up the stairs behind Jeff to get dressed to go to the hospital. In weaving the renovations and photograph together in my mind I realized something—we didn't even have an upstairs bedroom at the time I was writing about. Yet I still clearly see myself walking up those stairs after the phone call from the intensive care unit. After hearing Dr. Schacter, I realized there was no way to know whether or not the way I remembered the events of 1986 was correct, and at that moment I let go of the sense of obligation I'd had about recounting events exactly as they happened. Originally I had hoped that Jeff would fact-check the manuscript for me, but I eventually decided I did not want him to fix the facts. We might disagree on how or when things happened, and then what would I do? How could we know who was right? In the end I decided this was my story to tell, and I wrote it as I remembered it. The nurse moved back just a little, and the creative mother-writer stepped forward and took over. These are my truths.

I am sometimes surprised now when I read the words on these pages, because in putting the memories on paper I've been able to release them from my memory bank. Dr. Schacter writes that disclosing difficult experiences to others or writing them down can have profoundly positive psychological effects. Now that my memories are on paper, I've found that thoughts from Sarah's first year don't rattle around inside my skull any more. When I look at Sarah, I see her not as the preemie she was but as the gracious young woman she is today who still has the same fire, spirit, and charm that she showed in the first year of her life.

In July of 2004 I attended a LaScala family reunion. There were nearly a hundred people at a family camp on the Connecticut River, and there was no question that we were descendents of the same two people. Sarah fit in perfectly. With her olive skin and dark hair she looks more like an Italian LaScala than a Swedish Blomstedt. But then again, her eyes are green, and when you sit her next to Jeff's sister Martha, there are undeniable similarities. As I watched groups being gathered for photographs, it was hard to believe how lonely I was the year Sarah was born. My father was one of nine children, and I was approximately number seven of the thirty-six grandchildren. Most of these people lived within fifty miles of us in 1986. I believe now that I could have asked any one of them for help, but I never did.

I wonder if my isolation the year Sarah was born was more self-imposed than real. There were many people who wanted to help Jeff and Willie and me, but I didn't know what to ask for. More time with Sarah? More time with Willie? Who could have given me that? I didn't have time for visitors, and I didn't want to explain Sarah's condition to people on the phone each day. Her progress was too slow, and there wasn't much change to report from one day to the next. There certainly was not much good news, and I couldn't bear to rehash the parts that scared me.

So my loneliness wasn't from a lack of people in my life. I had a few new friends, far-away old friends, family only two hours away. I just didn't know how to begin the asking. What was striking about the LaScala reunion was that the aunts, uncles, and cousins were meeting Sarah for the first time, and her prematurity was still very real to them. It was a step back in time for me to witness their reactions to her, because, of course, the friends and family who have had relationships with Sarah over the last eighteen years have moved beyond the wonder of her survival. It was satisfying for me, as I finished writing about the year when Sarah was a baby, to be with people who reminded me of why I had been compelled to write this story in the first place.

At the family reunion I heard bits and pieces about people's lives: stories of cousins who survived cancer and some who did not; stories of car accidents, divorces, heart problems, anxiety, depression and all the things you'd expect to hear if you interviewed one hundred people who ranged from eight weeks to eighty years of age. On the day of the reunion Sarah's life story was no more or less important than any one else's. In the bigger world there are countless families of premature babies who can tell their own variations on a story like Sarah's, and in some ways I feel presumptuous telling this one. But Sarah is a remarkable example of survival, and my family happens to be incredibly fortunate to have her with us. I think as humans we derive hope from such stories, and we learn from them.

I had a number of goals in writing this book. I wanted to record the details of Sarah's year so I could remember and she could know the journey she took as a tiny baby.

Because I am a nurse, I wanted to illustrate for nurses and physicians how they / we look from the patient's and the family's perspective. I want nurses to see how important a moment of their time can be to a frightened patient. I want neonatologists and pediatric intensivists to look at Sarah's doctors and see how they fit in the picture as caregivers.

Another reason for sharing Sarah's story is to show an appreciation for the complexity of the human body. It took the combination of many minds, ever-emerging technology, and incredible luck to save Sarah's life. It also took more than five hundred thousand dollars (valued at 1986 rates) to pay for what would have been an economical fifteen weeks in my uterus.

Finally, I have two wishes. I hope the parents of premature babies find support and encouragement in the story of Sarah's successes. I also hope readers learn how to reach out to a sister, daughter, friend, or co-worker whose normal pregnancy is unexpectedly interrupted and who finds herself in the hospital with a baby born too soon.

ACKNOWLEDGMENTS

I wish I could sprinkle my gratitude around the country like pixie dust, in the same way Sarah's smile touched the doctors and nurses at her first birthday party. My thank-you list begins with nurse-midwife Liza Ramlow, who said to me one day when we were working together at Pioneer Women's Health, "Susan, do you want to join a writing group meeting at my house this evening?" Jan Frazier, the leader of that group, was the first reader of this book many years later, and she brought kindness and generosity to her writing groups and her critiquing. Sue Slavin, who babysat for Willie back in 1986, believed in this book without having read a word of it and arranged for me to meet friends who sent me to Haley's. The team work of editor and publisher Marcia Gagliardi, copy-editor Mary-Ann Palmieri, and editor Jane Gagliardi made me a better writer, and bg Thurston read and re-read with a keen eye. Abigail Rorer designed the cover with simplicity and elegance.

In the friends department much appreciation goes to Ginny Chandler, my mentor and dear friend, who called from Salt Lake City many times in 1986, then asked me to read early versions of this book to her nursing classes at UMass fifteen years later. My book group, including Sally, Terry, Sheila, Ginny, and Margo; my walking friends Doff and Emily; and my family planning colleagues Barbara, Jan, and Barbara were early readers and supporters who said all the right things often enough to keep me going. Many of our 1986 friends didn't make it into the story, but Susan Fish, the Rosses, Schwantes, Halls, Hills, Tiffanys, Ehrets, Coghlans, Hysons, Pachners, Civellos, Chester-McKusicks, Elstner-Bagalios, and Kendall-Shermans called us from near and far, babysat for Willie, brought casseroles to our kitchen, and ensured our nutritional and emotional survival. Lynda Hodsdon deserves the Medal of Honor for her great heart, her flexibility in times of need, and for creating a warm, safe, home-away-from-home for my children.

My mom, dad, and sisters helped out by knitting booties, sewing preemie-sized dresses and quilts, and caring for Willie over the year of Sarah's hospitalization; Jeff's brothers and sisters rooted for Sarah long-distance and sent Muz and Puz as the cavalry to rescue us over and over again. Because they are my professional family, I include here my co-workers at Deerfield Academy who helped me visualize the cover, asked about the book often enough to let me know they cared about it, and gave me Wednesdays off to finish it.

The list of Sarah's caregivers is long, and I'm sure I remember only a few of the people who touched her life. I can't begin to thank Hugh Roberts, our intrepid, unflappable pediatrician. He stood at the ready during Sarah's first year and continued as my children's ever-reliable doctor for the next sixteen years. Dr. Barbara Stechenberg devoted many hours to Sarah in 1986 and managed to wrap her intelligence and expertise in great warmth. I am indebted to the specialists and staff of Baystate's neonatal intensive care unit, including Dr. Bhavesh Shah and the neonatologists, and Beverly Siano and the nurses. An equal measure of gratitude goes to Dr. Stephen Lieberman and the staff of the pediatric intensive care unit. The entire Franklin Medical Center gave so much to us in 1986—many thanks to everyone who took care of Sarah and gave a generous measure of TLC to "Doctor B."

My final appreciation goes to my dear family, Jeff, Will, and Sarah, for allowing me to turn a year of their lives into the words on these pages.

ABOUT THE AUTHOR

Susan LaScala is the Director of Clinical Services at the Deerfield Academy Health Center. She has been a nurse practitioner for twenty-five years and a writer of stories, essays, and political commentary. She lives on Barton Cove in Gill, Massachusetts with two cats, one dog, and her husband, Jeffrey Blomstedt. Their two children return to the nest intermittently. Will attends Dartmouth College, and Sarah is a student at Bates College in Lewiston, Maine.

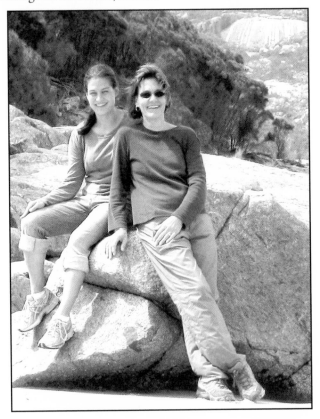

Susan LaScala and her daughter, Sarah Blomstedt

INDEX

breast milk 34, 41, 58, 77, 78, 108, 115, 118, 131, 144, 145, 168
breast pump 33, 121
bulldog clamp 238

C

Caesarean 17, 18, 59
caffeine 130
Canden (author's friend) 191
candida 64, 66, 109, 186, 187, 195
candidemia 68
catheter 60, 180, 194, 202, 206, 219, 233, 235, 241, 242, 243
central line 188, 194, 199, 205, 224, 227, 228, 229, 236, 238, 240, 241, 248
cervix 9, 17, 18
Chadds Ford 158, 160, 161, 244
chorioamnionitis 15, 25
Citrobacter 224
Connecticut River 48, 79, 191, 222
contractions 9, 10, 12, 17, 22
coworkers. *See* Jean, Maria, Sarah
creatinine 203, 212
Crisis Theory 165, 168
Crystal (patient with brain injury) 60, 61

D

Dad (author's father-in-law) 136, 157-160, 164. *See also* Puz
Dad (author's) 11, 42, 47, 48, 153. *See also* Grandpa
Danielle (author's friend) 50
Darlene (nurse) 89, 106, 119
David (nurse) x, 45, 57, 59, 67, 68, 73, 74, 75, 89, 96, 104, 123, 150, 172, 173, 190, 253

Decadron 110, 115
Deedy (author's friend) 156, 157, 223, 224
Demerol 25, 26, 28
dialysis 6, 16, 29, 84, 211, 212, 213, 215, 249
Dilantin 200
director of the pediatric ICU 211
due date 5, 8, 17, 30, 127

E

Ed (author's relative) 158
Eileen (author's friend) 189, 190, 191, 193, 194, 210, 220, 221
Elaine (author's relative) 42, 156, 157, 223
electrolytes 59, 203
electrolyte solution 143
Ellen (patient with leukemia) 165, 166
EMT 10
endotracheal tube 2, 23, 45, 54, 75, 90, 104, 108, 114, 123, 199, 201, 217, 229. *See also* ET tube
epidural blood patch 38
Eric (author's relative) 158, 244
ET tube 52, 68, 74, 75, 76, 77, 88, 96, 105, 106, 107, 109, 110, 113, 115, 218. *See also* endotracheal tube
extubation 104, 105, 107-111, 114, 115, 117, 119, 123, 143, 223, 230, 232

F

family planning 30, 46, 49, 188
fetus 14, 16, 17, 41, 53, 59, 62

fever 23, 25, 67, 140-142, 144, 173,
    175, 222, 224, 225, 237, 238
5-fluorocytosine 186
formula 115, 120, 123, 131, 133,
    156, 167, 168, 174, 193, 233
Franklin Medical Center 9, 92, 117,
    126, 127, 143, 144, 239, 240,
    242, 247, 250
friends. *See* Adrienne, Al, Anne,
    Barbara, Becky, Canden,
    Danielle, Deedy, Eileen,
    George, Ginny, Gordie,
    Jim, Jon, Kate, Lea, Lisa,
    Nathaniel, Patrick, Phil,
    Sarah
fungus 184, 224

G
Gayle (nurse) 37, 38, 40
gentamicin 103, 225
George (author's friend) 43
Ginny (author's friend) 96
glucose 57, 124
Gordie (author's friend) 97, 100
grading system, author's 3, 11, 12,
    17, 19, 38, 126, 185
Grandma (author's mother) 11, 32,
    48, 69, 134, 168, 222, 251
Grandpa (author's father) 11, 69,
    222, 223

H
"Hazards of Immobility" 168
headache 36, 38, 39, 40, 157
Health Choice 135
hemangioma x, 106, 183, 248
Hibiclens 95
HMO 135
Hugh. *See* Roberts, Hugh

hyperalimentation 98
hyperemesis 46

I
immunizations 171, 173, 180, 224
Indocin 62, 63, 66, 67, 68
internist 157
interns 15, 205, 251
intravenous access 205
    corticosteroids 60
    Decadron 11. *See also* IV
        Decadron
    fluid 57. *See also* IV fluid(s)
    line 123, 228. *See also* IV
    nutrition 76
    therapy 187. *See also* IV
        therapy
intubation 23, 105, 109, 113-115,
    195, 200, 201
IV 1, 2, 27, 36, 38, 41, 56, 57, 64,
    67, 85-88, 90, 124, 149, 186,
    187, 193, 199, 205, 207, 217,
    225, 227, 235, 238, 241
IV antibiotics 35, 232
    bag 27, 36
    board 88, 217
    Decadron 115. *See also*
        intravenous Decadron
    dressing 240
    feedings 76, 98
    fluid(s) 57, 87, 199, 202. *See
        also* intravenous fluid
    insertion 195
    medication 24
    medication bag 227
    medicine 25, 188
    placements 182
    pole 37, 61, 145
    port 24

IV antibiotics (continued)
  pump 67, 86, 187, 215, 230
  sites 224, 241
  therapy 235, 236. *See also*
    intravenous therapy

J

Jackie (nurse) 89, 90, 123, 135
Jean (author's coworker) 30
Jeffrey (author's relative) 158, 244
Jill (nurse) 127, 128, 248
Jim (author's friend) 189, 190, 208,
    210, 211
Jon (author's friend) 50, 80
José (patient in NICU) 54, 55

K

Kate (author's friend) 43
Kathryn. See Limmer, Kathryn
kidney infection 184-189, 193-233,
    239
Klebsiella 224

L

labor 7, 9, 11, 12, 14, 15, 17, 18, 19,
    22, 25, 81, 248
Lauren (nurse) 74, 75, 89, 123, 253
Lea (author's friend) 177
light therapy 56
Limmer, Kathryn 242, 243
Lisa (author's friend) 80, 81, 82
Lorie (author's relative) 29, 147,
    155
Lynda (babysitter) 49-51, 79, 80,
    94, 112, 129, 130, 139, 143,
    155, 182, 186, 188, 233, 236,
    240, 242, 249, 254-256

M

Mae (author's relative) 158
Maria (author's coworker) 8
Marianne (nurse) 225-230, 233, 238
Martha (author's relative) 158, 262
McAuliffe, Christa 69
Meyer, Kathleen, 60, 66, 67, 68,
    252, 253
Mom (author's) 11, 42, 47, 48, 87,
    88, 167, 245, 246
monitor, heart 44, 74, 75, 96, 99,
    111, 120, 199, 206,
    213, 215, 217, 218
  screen 13, 219
mucous plug 14
Muz (author's mother-in-law) 46,
    131, 132, 138-143, 157-160,
    244, 245

N

Nathaniel (author's friend) 190,
    197, 210
NEC. *See* necrotizing enterocolitis
necrotizing enterocolitis 18
needle 13, 19, 24, 38, 39, 85, 86,
    150, 171, 180, 207
neonatal intensive care unit xii, 2.
    See also NICU
nephrologist 16, 66, 211, 212, 215
nephrostomy tubes 216, 219
NICU ix, 52, 56, 82, 92, 94, 103,
    110, 115, 147, 197, 198, 206,
    251-253. *See also* neonatal
    intensive care unit
NICU nurses 118, 127, 136, 156
  parents 117, 136
  staff 64, 95

ventilator 2, 23, 52, 56, 59, 63, 67,
68, 75, 81, 98, 105, 108, 109,
111, 113, 115, 122, 199,
206-208, 213, 218, 222, 225,
229, 257
ventilator alarms 74
hose 96
pressure 86

W

warmer 1, 2, 3, 22, 44, 56
Wesson Women's Hospital (origi-
nally Wesson Memorial
Hospital) 10, 12

X

X-ray 52, 76, 93, 108, 213, 219,223,
230, 232, 234, 259

Y

Yale-New Haven Hospital 94, 126,
165; *See also* pediatric ICU,
Yale-New Haven Hospital
and pediatric intensive
care unit, Yale-New Haven
Hospital
Yale University School of Medicine
159, 161
yeast ix, 63, 66, 181